Don Barrett

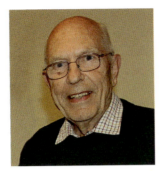

Originally hailing from Cambridge and a metallurgist by profession, Don, and his wife Lesley, moved to Addingham in 1995, particularly because of the great scenic walking country all around.

Joining the Addingham Civic Society ('ACS', he is now its Vice President) led to him meeting Arnold Pacey and Kate Mason, resulting in an interest in local history which, together with his love of nature, also gave purpose to his photography.

A long term computer geek, he used desk-top publishing to produce the ACS Newsletter for several years and has had a hand in the publication of their recent books (listed at the back), as editor, co-author and/or publisher.

This book combines most of these interests but particularly his love of walking, Addingham and the great outdoors.

Cover: Beamsley Beacon from a Moorside stile (now replaced by a gate - Walk 5)

Walks Around Addingham

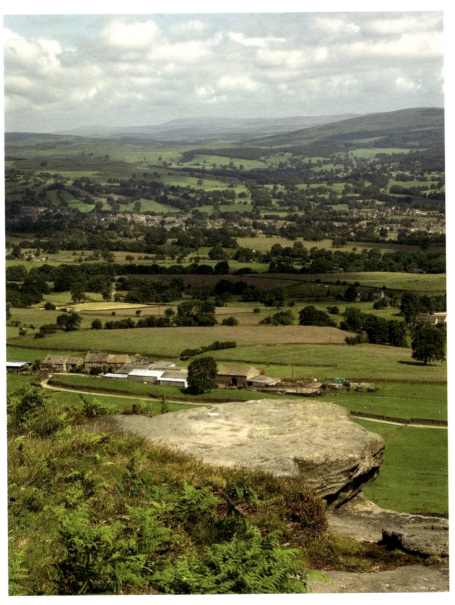

Addingham, in the mid-distance, from The Piper's Stone (Walk 5). Wharfedale stretches away to the north-west with Great Whernside and Buckden Pike on the skyline

Walks Around Addingham

A collection of circular walks of various lengths, all starting in the village of Addingham, West Yorkshire

Don Barrett

First published 2018 by Addingham Civic Society

Revision 1

c/o The Old School, Main Street, Addingham LS29 0NG

email: info@addinghamcivicsociety.co.uk

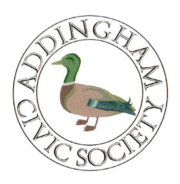

Copyright © 2018 Don Barrett

All rights reserved

ISBN: 9781980417323

Acknowledgements

The author's grateful thanks are due to all the people who have given help and encouragement with this project but especially the following, without whom the book would not be what it is:-

Alison Armstrong for her *'Country Walks Around Addingham'* which was the inspiration for, and the basis of, this book; **Jonathan White** for keeping me company while walking the walks and for all his helpful advice and comments; **Prof. Rick Battarbee (**and **Will Varley)** of the Addingham Environment Group for their geological and ecological information and other help; **Anne Hodgson** for the benefit of her extensive local walking knowledge and experience; **Arnold Pacey** and the late **Kate Mason** (personally and through their books) for historical information.

All remaining errors or omissions are entirely the author's responsibility - please send corrections and comments to him (email: don@addingham.info). Any resulting updates will be noted on the web page (addingham.info/walks)

Illustrations:
All photographs (except where indicated) by the author
Cartoon on page 9 by **Ken Birch**
Drawings on pages 37, 44 & 68 by **Alison Armstrong**
Drawings on pages 35 & 59 by **Arnold Pacey**
Mapping data licensed from Ordnance Survey © Crown Copyright 2018, licence No. CS-47311-B3T9X7.

Don Barrett
Addingham
March 2018

Map showing all the walks

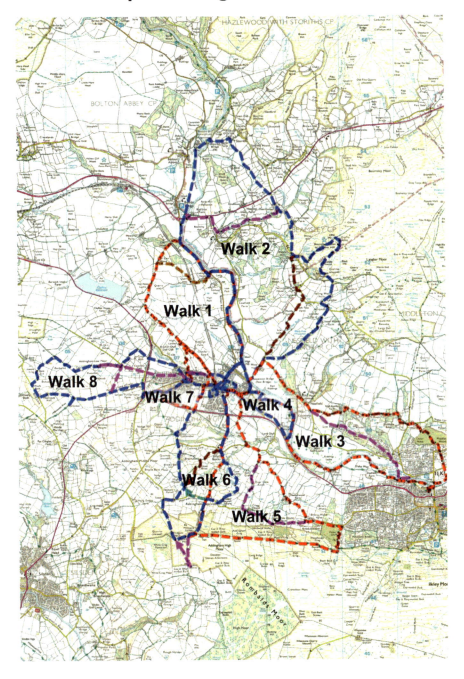

Contents

	Page
Introduction	1
Walking the Walks	7
Walk 1: Highfield, Lob Wood and The River Wharfe	11
Walk 2: Beamsley Beacon and Bolton Abbey	17
Walk 3: Ilkley and back via Nesfield, Middleton & the Dales Way	23
Walk 4: The Blue Plaques Trail	29
Walk 5: Netherwood House, Heber's Ghyll and the Moor Edge	41
Walk 6: Moorside and Millstones	49
Walk 7: Southfield, Marchup & High Laithe	57
Walk 8: Pre-Historic Addingham: Counter Hill and Round Dykes	63

Preface

Villages in Yorkshire, and indeed in the whole of England, are criss-crossed by public footpaths. Some date back to Medieval times and before, others are more recent, created to connect farms and villages as the old common fields were enclosed and privatised in the 18th and 19th centuries.

Today, since the 1949 National Parks and Access to the Countryside Act, most are protected as public rights of way, and these countryside paths are used not so much for essential journeys to work or school but for leisure. Old footpaths have been interconnected in imaginative ways to create networks of local walks, as Don Barrett has done in this volume.

This book has its origins in Alison Armstrong's booklet *'Country walks around Addingham, a landscape through history'* first published in 1992. The text differed from many collections of local walks by pointing out and explaining features of geological and archaeological interest along the way.

In this new collection of Addingham walks, Don has, in a masterly way, built upon Alison's legacy; updating and modifying a number of her original walks and creating new ones, including three much longer walks that stray well beyond the parish boundary. They are designed to take in much of the striking mid-Wharfedale landscape around Addingham and all the walks are succinctly described and beautifully illustrated.

This volume is an excellent addition to our village literature and I'm sure it will prove to be a very popular guide for both residents and visitors alike. It should cater for walkers of all persuasions, whether looking for healthy exercise, stunning landscapes, natural history or a combination of all three. Moreover they all start and finish close to a village public house!

Rick Battarbee

Addingham Environment Group
& University College London

Introduction

Addingham is an excellent base from which to walk, being in the valley of the River Wharfe but having the hill Beamsley Beacon to the north and the escarpment up to Rombald's Moor to the south. The routes chosen radiate out from the village; north to Bolton Abbey, east to Ilkley, south to Rombald's Moor, west to Counter Hill and to points in between, including two walks mainly within the village itself.

The inspiration for this book came from Alison Armstrong's book *'Country Walks Around Addingham'* but this author has expanded on her ideas by extending the walks further outside the Parish of Addingham, well into the beautiful surrounding countryside.

The area has an extensive network of public footpaths, many of them hundreds of years old, so there is plenty of opportunity to explore new country.

Addingham Village

Addingham is in the Metropolitan District of Bradford, between Ilkley and Skipton, close to the southern boundary of the Yorkshire Dales National Park and the Nidderdale Area of Outstanding Natural Beauty (AONB) which adjoins the eastern boundary of the National Park and extends to the far side of the River Wharfe in the vicinity of the village and towards Ilkley.

The Dales Way and the Dales High Way long distance paths pass through the village, as well as the Bradford Millennium Way circuit round the city. Parts of these are used on the walks in this book.

There is much evidence of pre-historic activity in the area (this is a feature on Walks 5 & 8), followed by the Romans who built a road through the edge of the modern village (Walks 6 & 8). The first written record referred to Archbishop Wulfere of York taking refuge here in AD 879 (Walk 4) but, from being a small farming community, the village was transformed into a busy textile mill village by the Industrial Revolution in the 19th century (Walk 4), with five mills and many other weaving sheds and related works being set up, plus a sawmill and five public houses.

Now, industry has largely gone and the village is home to a mainly commuter and retirement community, but with an active social life.

The Countryside and Geology around Addingham

Wharfedale is a glaciated valley, with the characteristic U shape, formed by the Wharfedale Glacier during the ice ages which, in this area, cut through ancient sandstone rock with interbedded softer shales. This sandstone, notably the coarse 'Addingham Edge Grit', was formed when a huge river delta covered the area about 315 million years ago. The rock contains fossil impressions of tropical plants which were buried in the sands of the delta and it forms outcrops on Rombald's Moor to the south (Walks 5 & 6) and Beamsley Beacon to the north (Walk 2).

The slopes below the moors are characterised by landslips where sandstones overlying weaker shales collapsed on the steep slopes, following the melting of the ice. Land slippage is clearly visible on Walk 6. The meltwater flowing beneath the margins of the retreating ice also cut channels which can still be seen at Cat Steps and below Gildersber (Walk 6) and near Storiths (Walks 1 and 2).

A conspicuous landscape feature on the valley floor is the flat-topped gravel terraces which form steep bluffs along the river (Walks 1 & 2). Towards the end of the last glacial period, about 15,000 years ago, the river flowed at a higher level than today, carrying large volumes of meltwater to Glacial Lake Humber, a huge lake dammed by ice in the North Sea. As the ice melted, the lake was drained and the river cut down through previously deposited layers of gravel, leaving them standing as terraces above the present day level of the river. White limestone pebbles, carried by ice from higher up the valley, may be found where the river has eroded these terraces. In the 18th and early 19th centuries, limestone boulders were gathered from the river and burnt to make lime, which is used to improve agricultural soils and to make mortar for building.

When the river water levels are low, it is noticeable how the sandstone rocks in the river bed stand on end towards Farfield but are nearly horizontal as High Mill is approached. These rocks were pushed up into a huge fold by movements in the earth's crust 270 million years ago. The top of this fold has now been eroded away, exposing Carboniferous limestone at its core which extends from Bolton Abbey to nearby Haw Pike and has enabled a delightful collection of lime-loving wild flowers to grow at Bolton Abbey Station.

Flora and Fauna

There are two main types of land in the area covered by these walks: acid heather moorland on the high ground and grassland of varying quality below the moors. There is also some woodland (Walks 1 & 3) and riverine habitat (Walks 1 & 2). The following notes highlight some of the more abundant species but good field guides will help identify the many other plants and animals to be seen.

Moorland:

The high moorland vegetation is dominated by ling (common heather) which produces the lovely purple haze over the hills in August. There is also bell heather in the drier areas, cross-leaved heath in wetter patches, heath bedstraw, and large amounts of bilberry with its upright green stems and small black berries in the autumn (they are tasty but it takes a lot of picking to make a meal!). In the wetter areas are rushes and cotton grass but bracken tends to dominate the lower, better drained, slopes.

The moors around Beamsley Beacon (Walk 2) are part of the Duke of Devonshire's Bolton Abbey Estate and are managed for grouse shooting which takes place after the 'Glorious' 12th of August.

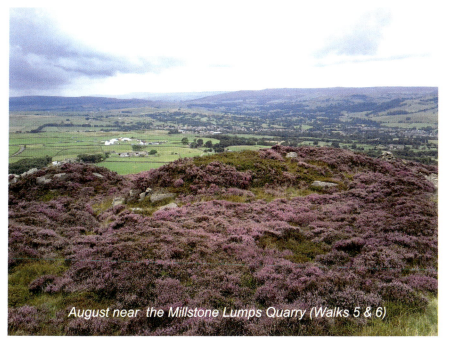
August near the Millstone Lumps Quarry (Walks 5 & 6)

In order to encourage the new heather shoots which the grouse enjoy, the moors are a patchwork of different colours where there has been rotational burning of the old growth during the winter.

The most obvious birds here are the Red Grouse, with its distinctive 'Go-back!' calls, which survive on the moors year-round, but the Red Kite, with its distinctive shape (photo overleaf), is now very often seen soaring above. Their numbers are increasing well following the very successful re-introduction releases at nearby

Harewood House and elsewhere. Other birds that you may see on the high ground include the little Meadow Pipit, Golden Plover and, possibly, Merlin.

Badgers like to make their setts on the slopes among the bracken and sometimes share them with fox families.

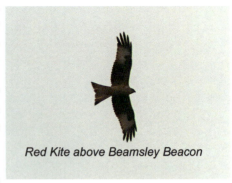
Red Kite above Beamsley Beacon

Grassland:

Many of the lower and more level meadows and pastures have been 'improved' by ploughing and re-seeding with tough ryegrass mixtures. This gives better quality grazing and good crops for silage but results in a mono-culture devoid of the wild flowers present in traditionally managed hay meadows. However, some of the rougher meadows have escaped this 'improvement' and areas such as Steg Holes (Walk 6) are consequently a mass of colour, as is the village nature reserve at Marchup Ghyll (Walks 7 & 8).

In Spring there are ragged robin, with its pink spidery petals, and cuckoo flower (milkmaids) in the wetter areas, with meadow buttercup, betony and even common spotted orchids, among many others, flowering in summer. The bases of dry-stone walls and roadside verges are often protected from disturbance and blue meadow cranesbill, aniseed-scented sweet cicely, foxglove and giant bellflower take advantage of this.

The dominant grassland fauna is the sheep! In fact, there are few other farm animals in this area though cattle are sometimes seen, including at Gildersber (Walk 6) and on the riverside meadows (Walks 1 & 2, photo below).

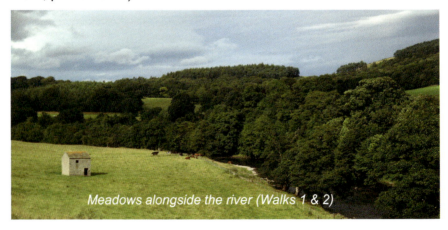
Meadows alongside the river (Walks 1 & 2)

Spring starts, in my opinion, when the warbling of the curlew is first heard over the meadows in February or March and these large birds are common here, though decreasing nationally. They are joined by oystercatchers, with their piercing whistles, and, in the nesting season, lapwing (or peewit/tewit) will swoop and shout at intruders, animal or human, getting too near their nest. Like the curlew, they are ground-nesting and therefore very vulnerable to predation and disturbance. Another meadow bird, the skylark, can often be heard, trilling as it ascends to the heights.

Rivers and Becks:

The riverside is a feature on Walks 1 & 2 and there are many becks on the other walks. Alder is a tree that revels in having its feet wet but there are a number of other trees, including oak, sycamore, goat willow and horse chestnut along the banks. Grazing limits the ground flora but, where protected from the sheep, coltsfoot, lesser celandine and butterbur will be seen early in the year with, later, giant bellflower, meadowsweet and, also sweet smelling but invasive, Himalayan balsam. The yellow flowers of golden saxifrage are common in the becks.

Some of the birds seen along the Wharfe are shown below, including the flamboyant mandarin duck which is now well established in the area, particularly around Bolton Abbey. Others include the grey wagtail, goosander and, of course, mallard, with black-headed gulls

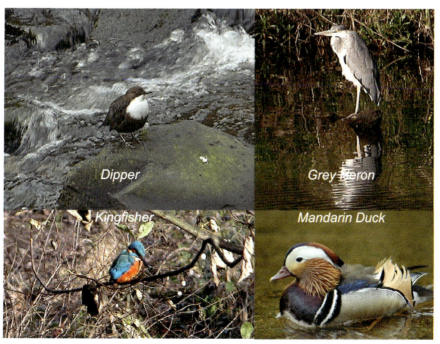

from the well-established gullery on Barden Moor, and cormorants, joining them.

Otters have been reported, now that the predatory mink are less numerous, and they will prey upon the alien signal crayfish (which has now almost replaced the native white clawed species). The Wharfe river itself has brown trout and grayling although trout are now rare in the becks.

Woodland:

Compared to the generally sparse woodland cover in the Dales National Park, there *are* areas of woodland around here and these walks include several of them, notably, Lob Wood (Walk 1) and Middleton Woods (Walk 3). There are also smaller areas at Marchup Ghyll (Walks 7 & 8) and Lumb Ghyll (Walk 5). Just north of Walk 2 is the large woodland area of the Strid Woods, Bolton Abbey Estate.

All these are mixed deciduous woods, mainly of oak, sycamore, alder, beech and ash - the latter now almost certainly doomed by the spread of Ash Dieback Disease. Fortunately, perhaps, ash does not dominate here as it tends to on the limestone country further north so the effect might not be quite so devastating as it is likely to be there.

All the above woods are carpeted with bluebells in the spring, together with wood anemones, wild arum, wild garlic (ransoms) and red campion. When the canopy closes over, these die back in the gloom and only plants which can tolerate low light, like ferns, green the woodland floor.

Numerous birds frequent woodland, of course, but they can be hard to see up in the canopy. However, the loud drumming of the great spotted woodpecker cannot be missed and both grey nuthatches

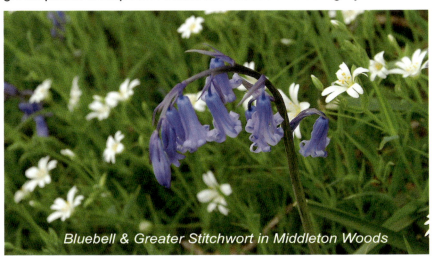
Bluebell & Greater Stitchwort in Middleton Woods

and brown tree creepers can be seen on the trunks, searching for grubs.

Walking the Walks

The map at the front of the book shows all the walks and how they are arranged, radiating out from the village but all starting and finishing on Main Street, Addingham.

The detailed descriptions which now follow start with the distances and height gain, followed by a summary of the walk to help you decide which one to choose, a walk route map, height profile to show the gentle bits and then step by step directions to guide walkers on their way. These are interspersed with background information and many photographs to add interest to the walk.

All these walks are suitable for people of average fitness but, since Addingham is near the bottom of the valley, all involve some, generally fairly gentle, uphill walking. The highest points are Beamsley Beacon (Walk 2) and Rombald's Moor (Walks 5 & 6) which are about 1200ft (400m) above sea level whereas the start points on Main Street are at about 270ft (89m) above sea level, so these three walks are the most strenuous. Most of the going is on paths, tracks or grassy meadows but the Millstones Quarry (Walks 5 & 6) and the 'Rocky Road' down Beamsley Beacon (Walk 2) are rougher.

There are numerous stone wall stiles on the walks and some are rather high, demanding reasonable agility, particularly for those with short legs - leaders of groups may need to bear this in mind when estimating the time required. We do not include estimates of how long the walks will take because this varies so much from group to group, depending not only on their walking speed but also on the number of walkers in the group and the amount of time taken admiring the view, taking photographs, observing wildlife or having rests and refreshment.

The lengths of the walks vary from about 3 to 9 miles, but all include short cuts and options to enable walkers to tailor their outing to suit themselves, their fitness, and the time available. **Note that, in the descriptions and maps, the short-cuts are colour coded to differentiate them from the main routes. If you are walking the main (full) route just ignore the coloured paragraphs.**

Navigation

The directions, in conjunction with the route map, should enable walkers to find their way without trouble, particularly as clear landmarks such as Beamsley Beacon to the north, and The Moorside (up to Rombald's Moor) to the south, are often visible to aid orientation. Although the base of the route maps is the Ordnance Survey map, these have been scaled to fit the page and give maximum clarity. This means that the map scale varies from walk to walk, although the kilometre squares can be used as a guide. We recommend that all walkers carry a paper map (OS Explorer 297 or Landranger 104), and compass, to give an accurate idea of distance and position. The detailed information on these excellent maps will also add interest.

GPS Navigation

Those with mobile phones or tablets may find them useful to aid navigation. There are notes on this, and downloadable copies of the directions, on the village website: *addingham.info/walks*.

Other equipment

The best thing to take with you on any walk is a good dollop of common sense! With this in hand there is no need to over-emphasise 'health and safety', but remember that the weather can change quickly, it will always be **colder** on 'the tops', and may well be **muddy** underfoot, so dress **suitably**. Hey, it is Yorkshire, after all!

Of course, you walk entirely at your own risk and please obey The Countryside Code - leave no litter, leave gates as you found them and keep dogs on a short lead when near farm animals.

**Don't over-stretch yourself, just enjoy the walk!
With glorious country like that shown below on our doorstep who could not enjoy it?**

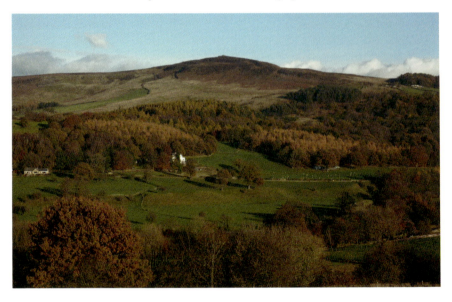

Beamsley Beacon from Farfield (Walk 1)

Walk 1: Highfield, Lob Wood and the riverside

The Walks

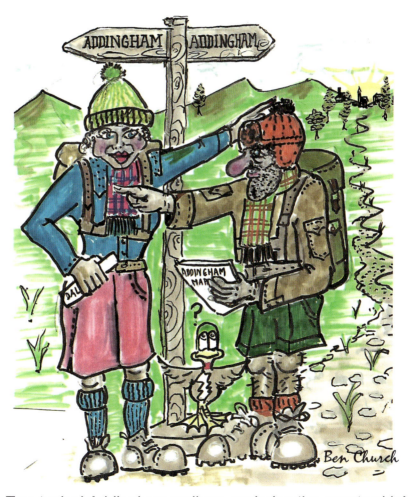

Two typical Addingham walkers exploring the countryside!

Walk 1: Highfield, Lob Wood and the riverside

Walk 1
Highfield, Lob Wood and The River Wharfe

Start: The Hen Pen Garden, Main Street, Addingham LS29 0NS, SE 077 498.
Alternative Start: Near Bolton Bridge SE 071 525 (see page 15).
Full walk: 4.5 miles (7.2km), height gain 584ft (190m).
Shorter walk: 4 miles (6.4km), height gain 584ft (190m).

Summary:

This is a fairly easy walk with lots of interesting features along the way, including fine views across to Beamsley Beacon (photo below) and up Wharfedale to Bolton Abbey and beyond, the dramatic (but almost hidden) Lob Wood railway viaduct, the ancient Farfield Friends' Meeting House, abundant wildlife and a lovely Dales Way river walk to finish. The route description includes an optional shorter link, which avoids the sometimes slippery steps and path in Lob Wood, and an alternative start point near Bolton Bridge.

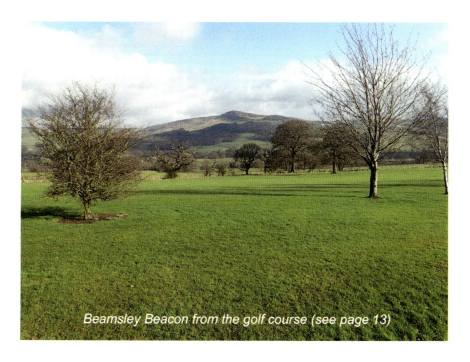

Beamsley Beacon from the golf course (see page 13)

Walk 1: Highfield, Lob Wood and the riverside

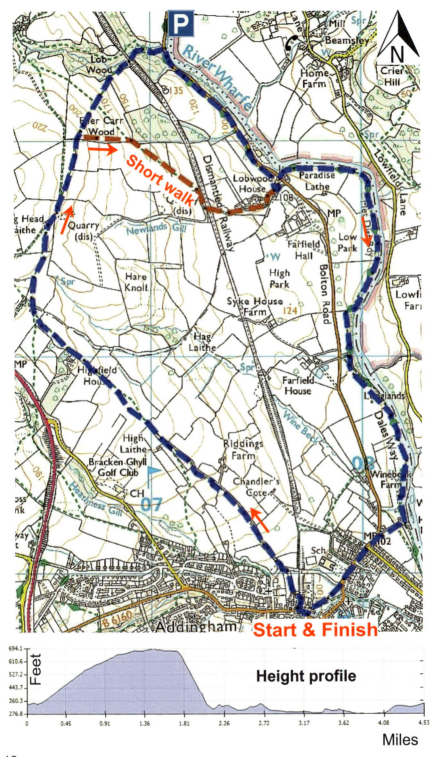

Walk 1: Highfield, Lob Wood and the riverside

The Walk

The walk begins at the **Hen Pen Garden**, where Main Street bends in the middle of Addingham village, and it is usually possible to park on Old Station Way almost opposite. After admiring the flowers in the garden (maintained by the Addingham Garden Friends volunteers), the route **goes up** the adjacent Sugar Hill and **left** on Back Beck Lane before turning **almost immediately righ**t (north) up Long Riddings Lane. On the end of the second house in the lane it is possible to see where there was a 'taking-in' door on the first floor which indicates that the occupants were once in the domestic textile industry. Here, yarn and cloth could be winched in and out of the loomshop above the living accommodation. After a short distance the path **leaves** the lane through a gate **on the left,** by a tree, just after the ruin of Low Laithe (previously called New Laithe - 'laithe' means barn or granary and this small barn had a threshing floor and mistal for six cows).

The path now goes gently **uphill** across meadowland beside the overgrown Long Riddings Lane, which was probably the road to the medieval open 'High Field'. The lane hedge is rich in tree species and is also a haven for wildlife. There are fine views back over Addingham and up to Addingham Moorside and Rombald's Moor from here.

After three fields, the ruin of High Laithe (18th century barn) is on the left (see Walk 7, p61, for details). The path now **crosses the golf course** (Bracken Ghyll Golf Club, watch out for flying balls!) and is marked by **coloured posts**. There are great views of Beamsley Beacon across the valley (see photo on page 11). After crossing the first fairway follow a mown path **(left)** and, after passing a stone hut, go **left** over a stile into the field beside Highfleld House, with its unusual large windows, which dates from about 1780. **Continue along**, left of the fairway, to the course boundary.

After leaving the golf course, **cross the field diagonally right** in front of Highfield Farm. This was formally called Hag Head and is a 'laithe-house' farm (a house and barn joined in one long-house) dating from about 1800. Cross to the wall stile **in the corner** of the field, with the serpentine medieval boundary ditch and bank of Addingham parish in the next field. **Continue** across a small valley and **up** to another wall stile, then **cross the field** to go round the end of the wall. Remains of ancient field barns belonging to Hag Head can be seen at this high point of the walk. The route **goes right** along a farm track but, after the metal gate, it **leaves** the track and **follows the wall on the right** to a wall stile in the **far right** corner of the field.

Walk 1: Highfield, Lob Wood and the riverside

At the stile, take time to enjoy a fine view (photo below) of Bolton Priory and the narrow old Bolton Bridge (beyond the modern road bridge), beneath the rocky summit of Simon's Seat. Medieval plough strips can be seen in the fields below. The curious 'nicks' in the hillside at Storiths across the valley are deep channels cut across the spur of the hill by meltwater flowing beneath the retreating ice at the end of the last ice age.

For the shorter walk turn right after this stile, steeply down the field, passing small delfs (pits or quarries) where Millstone Grit

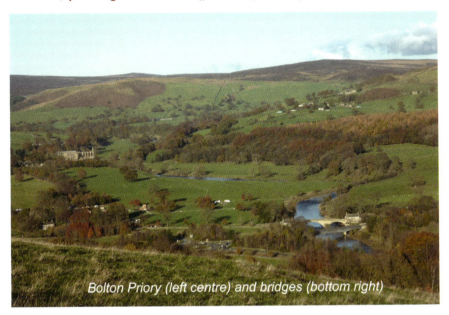
Bolton Priory (left centre) and bridges (bottom right)

sandstone has been taken, probably for wallstones. Go **right again** through a stile in the wall near the corner of Eller Carr Wood (the name indicates Elder trees growing on wet ground) and keep **diagonally downhill** toward the buildings. Cross another field, through the **gate** in the corner and **along the track** towards the Farfield Livery stables, going (left) through a gap where the railway line once crossed. The rear of Farfield Hall may be seen from the path, over to the right. It was enlarged about 1728 by Anthony Myers with the old 17th century house now incorporated at the west end. After walking **through the stables**, the route **goes right**, down the track closed to vehicles by large stones, to rejoin the route of the **longer walk** at the metal gate **(go to next page).**

The full walk continues diagonally down the pastures in the direction of Bolton Bridge, in the distance, to another **stile** near the **bottom corner** of the field and into Lob Wood. In the wood, the path

Walk 1: Highfield, Lob Wood and the riverside

initially **follows the wall** (right) but then turns **left** down **steep steps (which can be slippery)** before revealing the spectacular Lob Ghyll Viaduct (Bridge No.47) (photo below) which took the Ilkley to Skipton railway (built in 1888) on its way to Bolton Abbey Station. After going under the viaduct **(with care!)**, **the path bears right and down** through the mixed deciduous woodland (woodland is a rarity around Addingham - see Introduction) to **steps down** to the road **near Bolton Bridge**.

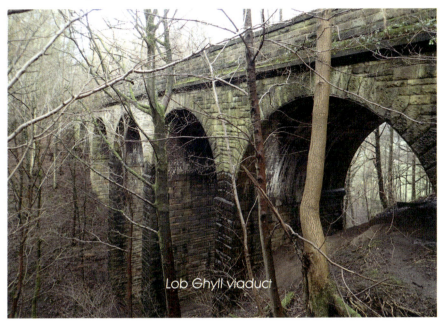
Lob Ghyll viaduct

This makes a good alternative start point for the walk; there is (limited) parking along the road and on the other side of the roundabout. **If starting from here**, Addingham provides ample places for refreshment at the halfway point of the walk.

The route goes **right,** up the road, **(take extra care on this steep, narrow, and busy stretch of road)** and **crosses** the road to a track about 150 metres up the hill.

After leaving the road, and now following the Dales Way (see Walk 3, p27, for details), **follow the wall** all the way to Farfield. Visible on the river bank across the road is the drab, but award winning, Lob Wood Pumping Station which pumps water from the Barden reservoirs, and the Wharfe, up to Chelker Reservoir until needed to provide water for the Bradford area. **Keep right** of the driveway and up to go **left at the metal gate** behind Farfield Cottages.

The shorter walk re-joins the longer walk here.

15

Walk 1: Highfield, Lob Wood and the riverside

The route now goes **left again,** behind the Farfield Meeting House, which is usually open and is well worth visiting (see Walk 4, p37, for details), before again reaching and crossing Bolton Road **(take care!)** and going down steps to join the river bank. The first field is called 'Paradise'(!) and Paradise Laithe at the top was formerly an 18th century aisled barn with its cart entrance leading to the grain threshing floor.

The path **continues along** this delightful stretch of river, popular with anglers (see the Introduction for details of the geology and nature), still following the Dales Way, along the **riverside,** across meadows and over stiles, for about 1½ miles (2½ km). The path leads to the caravan and chalet site before High Mill (photo right), which stands on the river beyond its long weir. In medieval times, the Lord of the Manor's water-powered corn mill stood here. Cloth fulling probably also once took place since the small field, now a car park behind, is called 'tenterlands', indicating the place where woven and fulled woollen cloth was stretched to dry on tenter hooks. The present mill buildings date from the late 18th and early 19th century when the old 17th century corn mill was extended for worsted, and later for silk spinning.

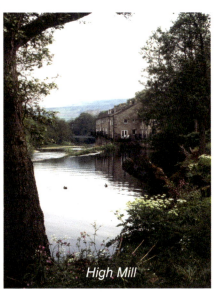
High Mill

After the chalets, **turn right up High Mill Lane.** The last house at the top has a classically designed datestone of 1812 and was probably built for the mill manager.

Turn left onto Bolton Road, cross Bark Lane and pass, on the right, the lofty Victorian dwellings of Springfield Mount and the Manse (c.1885) and then Addingham Primary School, much acclaimed for its design when built in 1979. After the school, **cross diagonally right,** over the cattle grid onto the track across Manor Garth with, to the left, the Rookery (see Walk 4, p32, for details). Ahead to the right is another row of cottages, two of which were originally used for weaving but subsequently housed the Mechanics' Institute and Library. Straight ahead is the Manor House (again, see Walk 4).

The walk finishes here, **back on Main Street.**

Walk 2
Beamsley Beacon and Bolton Abbey

Start and Finish: The Memorial Hall, Main Street, Addingham, LS29 0LZ, SE 079 497
The shortest walk is about 5½ miles (8.8km)
The medium walk is about 8¼ miles (13.2km)
The full walk is about 9 miles (14.4km)
Height gain: 1022ft (335m)

Summary:

    This is a great walk up Addingham's local hill and on to the ancient ruins of Bolton Priory, before a gentle return along the riverside stretch of the Dales Way. Although the full walk is about nine miles, and includes the climb up Beamsley Beacon, there are two shorter options detailed, and a number of other possibilities if using other starting points. However, the 360 degree panorama from the top of the Beacon, and the dramatic ruins of Bolton Priory, make the effort well worthwhile.

    Note that areas of the Bolton Abbey estate are closed for shooting on certain days during the autumn - check local information before heading out at that time.

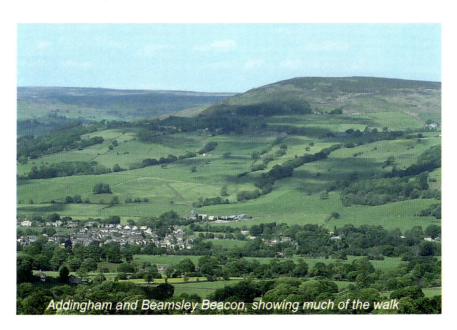
Addingham and Beamsley Beacon, showing much of the walk

Walk 2: Beamsley Beacon & Bolton Abbey

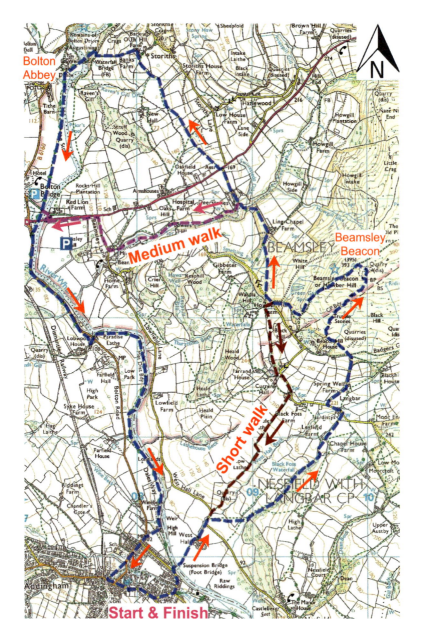

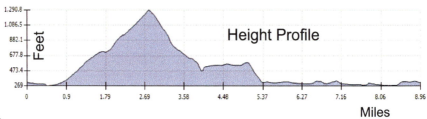

Walk 2: Beamsley Beacon & Bolton Abbey

The Walk

The walk starts from **The Memorial Hall**, Main Street, Addingham, opposite The Fleece, an inn dating back to the mid 18th century. **Turn right** and go down Main Street but **bear left** along Church Street. This was formerly Kirkgate and was the main road from Ilkley until lower Main Street (past the Cricket Club) was built in the 18th century as a turnpike road. The Church Street area is one of the three original clusters of buildings which eventually formed 'Long Addingham'; the others were around the Old School and around The Green and Moor Lane at the top of the village. Fir Cottage, on the left just before Parkinson's Fold, is considered the oldest house in Addingham because a Medieval hearth was found under the floor during renovation.

At the road junction, **cross** the road and go **left up** North Street to take the footpath, **right**, just after the bend (soon after the village information board) sp 'Dales Way'. Turn **right** partway down the steps and **cross the Suspension Bridge** (this bridge was built in 1935 to replace a wooden bridge built in 1896 but washed away in a flood. Prior to 1896 there was a ferry across the river at this point). **Continue** past the West Hall buildings to the (narrow) end of the footpath, go **right** through two gates and then **left** up the road.

The route continues **straight** at the road junction but **right** at the **wall stile** about 50m after this. From the stile go **diagonally left** across the field to the **right-hand** gate and then follow the wooded valley (do not cross the beck) up to Leyfield Farm. After the stile before the farm, **bear right** up the field then left to **cross** the front lawn of the farm, before turning **right**, up their drive to the road.

Go **left** along the road but turn **right** along a **track** (the **second** footpath), which turns uphill at the farm buildings. About 160m past the farm, **fork left** on a path up to the minor road. Turn **left** but **almost immediately** fork **right** on a grassy footpath toward the woods around Beacon Hill House. Cross a small beck and, when approaching the corner of the wall round the woods, **turn right** on a clear path towards the summit of Beamsley Beacon. The country is now heather moorland used for grouse shooting by the Bolton Abbey Estate (see notes in Introduction).

Keep following this path towards, but to the right of, the Beacon. The path bends left and then zigzags up to the huge cairn on the summit. The 'trig point' beside the cairn has two plaques: the top one mentions two nearby Bronze age burial mounds and the Napoleonic beacon which gave the hill its name. The lower plaque commemorates a WW2 plane crash which occurred on the Beacon (See 'Addingham in World War Two' for details). There is a tre-

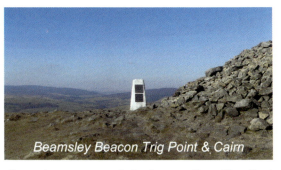
Beamsley Beacon Trig Point & Cairn

mendous 360° panorama from here, especially in weather like that shown in the photo, even though it was -2°C and blowing hard at the time! Enjoy the view, and use your map to identify the landmarks.

After a well-earned rest, **descend the rocky track** (left) but, towards the bottom, **turn right** on one of the paths which drop down to a wall round two small fields. **Follow** the wall down to the road.

For the shortest walk:
Cross over the road onto a driveway and take the footpath **left** (sp 'Currer Hall') just before the cattle grid. Bear **slightly left** to a wall stile and **continue** across fields, keeping the wall on the right. Go through a wood to the driveway of Currer Hall and **left** up to the road. **Turn right** down the road and after 150m turn **right** again over a cattle grid and then **left** down the track. Follow this track for about ½mile (800m) - it becomes narrow and sunken (and may be wet) after skirting round a house - down to a field and then the road. Straight ahead are West Hall and the Suspension Bridge crossed at the start.

For the longer walks:
Turn **right down the road** and after 80m take the footpath **right**, sp 'Harrogate Road 1¼ miles', across the moor to the farm track near Ling Chapel Farm. **Cross** the track diagonally and take the footpath, sp 'Deerstones'. Follow this path **down** through the wood before zigzagging down to, and across the bridge over Kex Beck (photo opposite) and then **up to** the houses at Deerstones hamlet.

For the medium walk:
When approaching the Deerstones houses, **turn left and follow the footpath**, sp 'Beamsley Lane', down through a wood above the stream (this is covered in bluebells in the season) and continue to follow the beck across fields. Just after a big black barn, **turn right** at the little humpback **bridge** (do not cross back over the beck), go **diagonally right** across fields to a footpath beside the old mill goit (stream) and then past the former Beamsley Mill, on the left, which it supplied, to the road. At the T-junction **turn right** and then **left** at the A59 Harrogate road. Take the cycleway/footpath on the **left**, go **right**

Walk 2: Beamsley Beacon & Bolton Abbey

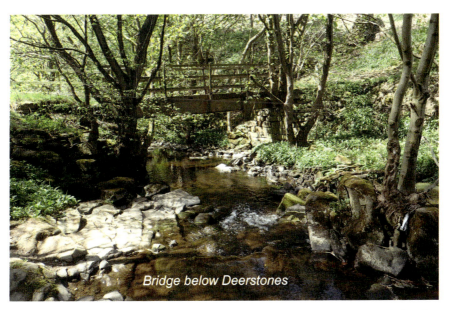
Bridge below Deerstones

under the road bridge and **left** over the old river bridge **to rejoin the full walk here (see p22).**

For the full walk:

Go **straight** through Deerstones hamlet, **cross** the main Harrogate Road **(with care!)** and take the footpath opposite. **Follow** the wall (on the left), ignore the crossing footpath but go **left over the wall stile** after about 700m and continue to follow the wall (now on the right) to Storiths hamlet.

After sp 'Priory Bridge ¼', **continue** through Storiths to a narrow track **(left)** down to the Priory, which can now be seen below (note that the name 'Bolton Abbey' is applied to the village but 'Bolton Priory' to the ruins and church).

At the bottom of the track **turn right**, where a fine view over the Priory, beautifully located beside a bend in the River Wharfe, can be admired (photo p22). **Then keep left** and follow the path to the river and across the wooden bridge (or risk the stepping stones!). This is your opportunity to go and look round the ruins and the church if you have time. The 'Hole in the wall' up to the left of the ruins leads to the village and tearooms.

The monastery was founded at Embsay in 1120 by the Augustinian order and moved to the present site, on land given by Lady Alice de Romille of Skipton Castle, in 1154. In the early 14th century Scottish raiders caused the temporary abandonment of the site and serious structural damage to the priory.

The nave of the abbey church was in use as a parish church

Walk 2: Beamsley Beacon & Bolton Abbey

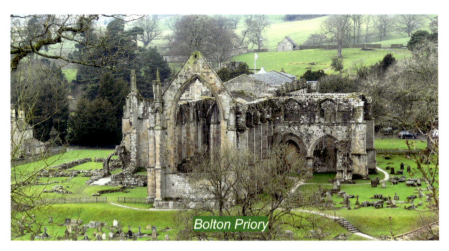
Bolton Priory

from about 1170 onwards and survived the Dissolution of the Monasteries which resulted in the end of the Priory in January 1540. The east end remains in ruins but the tower, begun in 1520 but left half-standing, was later given a bell-turret and converted into an entrance porch. It is still an active working church today.

The rest of the walk back to Addingham follows The Dales Way footpath. Returning from the Priory, follow the path, **right,** along the river bank **downstream** through the fields, passing the cricket ground behind the Devonshire Arms hotel on the right, **up to** a wall gate and **across** the road (the old Harrogate to Skipton Road, before the new bridge was built).

The medium walk (and Walk 1) join here.

Follow the Dales Way **down steps** beside the house, under the new bridge and then over a wooden bridge to the Bolton Road. **Turn left** up the road to go past the car parking area and up the hill **(take extra care on this steep, narrow, and busy stretch of road!). Cross** the road to a track about 150m after the parked cars and follow the wall for about ¾mile (1.2km), **keep right** of the driveway and go **left** at the metal gate behind Farfield Cottages. The path then goes **left** behind the ancient Friends' Meeting House (well worth visiting, see Walk 4), before **crossing** the road again **(take care!)** and down steps to join the river bank. The path continues for about 1½ miles (2.4km) along this delightful stretch of river, still following the Dales Way, (**see Walk 1 for details of this stretch**) to the caravan site and chalets at High Mill. Passing behind the mill note the Blue Plaque at the Dawson Crossley Field (see Walk 4). Continue along the river bank to the steps above the Suspension Bridge, up the steps to North Street, **left** down to Church Street, **right** towards Main Street and back to finish at the **Memorial Hall**.

Walk 3
Ilkley and back via Nesfield, Middleton & the Dales Way

Start & Finish: The Memorial Hall, Addingham Main Street, LS29 0LZ, SE 079 497
Full walk: 7¼ miles (11½ km)
Height gain: 360ft (109 m)
Shorter walk: 6 miles (9½ km)
Height gain: 162ft (53m)

Summary:

A gentle walk to Ilkley and back, good for a hot day as it is mostly shaded and wooded, but nice at any time. Convenient for a diversion into Ilkley for shopping or refreshment but also passes the Riverside pub which has a take-away food outlet. Ilkley would make an alternative start point and there is a shorter, lower, option.

Easy going, mainly across meadows and minor roads, returning along the riverside Dales Way.

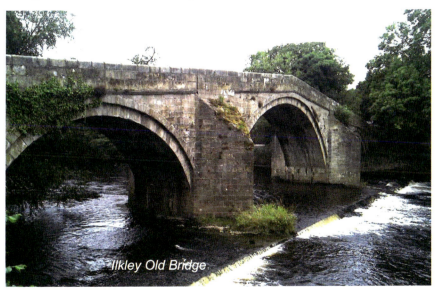

Ilkley Old Bridge

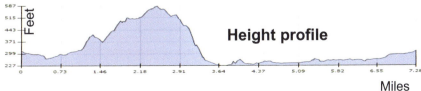

Height profile

Miles

Walk 3: Ilkley via Nesfield, Middleton & the Dales Way

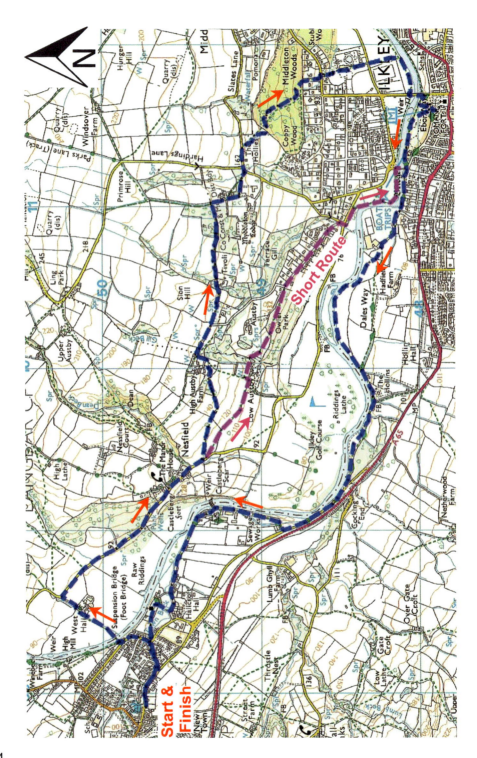

The Walk

The walk starts from **The Memorial Hall.** Turn **right** and go **down** Main Street but **bear left** into Church Street, formerly Kirkgate (the first part of this walk is the same as Walk 2, see p19 for details).

At the junction, cross the road and go **left up** North Street to take the **footpath right** just after the bend, soon after the village information board, sp 'Dales Way'. **Turn right** partway down the steps and **cross** the Suspension Bridge. **Continue** along the footpath, past the West Hall buildings, to the (narrow) end, **go right** through two gates and **left** up the road.

At the road junction, **turn right** and **follow** the road, which is narrow but has little traffic except for cyclists - it is on the Dales Cycleway. The road passes an old deerpark on the left, where the spaced out parkland trees can be clearly seen, before reaching the hamlet of Nesfield. On the right, opposite the Nesfield houses, is the tree-topped Castleberg Hillfort (photo below). This is said to date from the Iron Age but has never been properly excavated so could be earlier, maybe late Bronze Age. Up on the green to the left is a shelter which was used by the village postman as a rest place after his journey from Ilkley. It has now been renovated by the village (coffee, anyone?).

Continue past Nesfield, keeping **right** along the road, and just after an old stone bridge **turn left** up a farm track to a stile.

For the short route, take the **right-hand footpath** and, keeping the fence then the wall on your right, follow the path through three fields to Low Austby House.

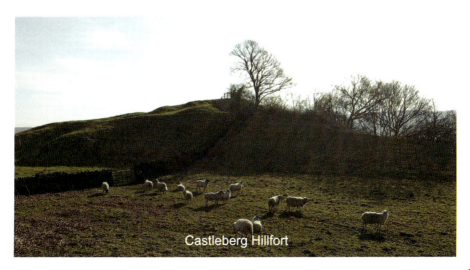
Castleberg Hillfort

Walk 3: Ilkley via Nesfield, Middleton & the Dales Way

In the field behind the house bear left and follow marker posts to a small bridge and into Spring Wood. The path drops down through the wood and then crosses a meadow, following the curve of the hill to Owler Park Wood. Both these woods are ablaze with bluebells in the spring. Continue through the wood and up to Owler Park Road.

Turn right through the houses to the bottom road. **Cross with care** and take the path along the river to the Old Bridge where the **full walk is rejoined (go to next page)**.

For the full walk, take the left-hand footpath to a **stile near the top** of the stone wall, below the wire fence. Follow the wall **round to the left** to another stile and High Austby Farm. There are fine views across to Rombald's Moor from here.

Follow the garden boundary across in front of the farmhouse to the stile right of the gate and **turn right** along the road, continuing **straight** on to the bridleway. After ½m (800 metres), in shady woods, **the road bends right** and continues downhill, following the track **left** past the entrances to Myddleton Lodge and Grange. The old lodge can be seen through trees on the right at the bend.

The Grade I listed Myddelton Lodge dates back to 1260 and was home for centuries to one of the town's most famous families, the Middletons. Myddelton has been a Catholic stronghold in the North of England since the 16th Century when the Middletons of Myddelton Lodge sustained the Catholic faith in and around Ilkley. Since 1922 Myddelton has been the site of a retreat centre, originally based in Myddelton Lodge and run by the Cross and Passion Fathers. In the mid 80s the Lodge was sold to the Diocese of Leeds and continued to run as a retreat centre until 2000.

After Myddleton Grange, turn left at the T-junction and then **right** along a minor road and go **right** over the fence stile after a gate. The path goes diagonally left across the field towards a large free-standing oak tree and then **over a stile** into Middleton Woods. Take the path **going left** to a large waymarked stone, bear right down the footpath and keep more or less straight and down flights of stone steps. Middleton Woods are a haven for numerous birds and, in late spring, are ablaze with bluebells (photo opposite) and Marsh Marigolds (Kingcups) in the wetter areas.

At the path junction, bear left over a wooden bridge and **along** the boardwalk, then keep **right** beside a large holly bush and down steps to the road. Turn left and then immediately right, down more steps to the park. Walk down the park, alongside the swimming pool, cross the road and continue down to the river.

Go right along the riverside path to the road bridge, up the steps to the road and cross the bridge. **The road ahead leads into**

Ilkley town centre for a diversion, or buses back to Addingham.

To continue the walk, go down the steps on the **right-hand** side of the road to the other (south) riverside path, into the **Riverside Gardens** and playground. After about 50m, climb up the grassy bank on the left to view the remains of **Ilkley Roman Fort** (Olicana), which has an information board. Continue along the riverside, past the Riverside pub (this supplies take-away food etc.) and toilets, to the Old Bridge. This 1675 bridge (photo on first page) was the only river crossing until the New Brook Street bridge (crossed earlier) was built in

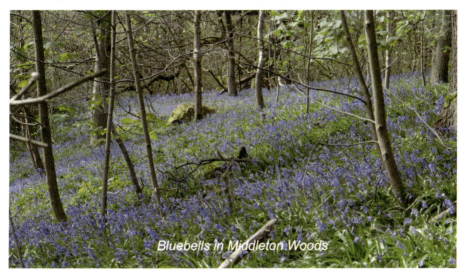
Bluebells in Middleton Woods

Victorian times.

The Old Bridge marks the start of the Dales Way which this walk now follows to Addingham. The Dales Way long distance footpath was founded in 1968 by Colin Speakman of Ilkley, in co-operation with the Ramblers' Association. It goes from Ilkley Old Bridge to Bowness-on-Windermere in the Lake District. Much of the 80 miles (128km) keeps to the valleys and riversides, for which the average walker may take from five to seven days. The path follows the River Wharfe through the Yorkshire Dales National Park, brushes with the Pennine Way, then goes down Dentdale into Cumbria to cross the River Lune and enter Lakeland.

The short route rejoins here.

From the Old Bridge, continue along the riverside to, and past, the tennis centre buildings but then **turn left** into a meadow and immediately **fork right** and follow the field edge to the **Woodland Walkway.** A sign indicates that there is no through way but it **is** now possible to walk through and rejoin the Dales Way after the wood. **Bear right** through the wood to continue along the riverbank.

Walk 3: Ilkley via Nesfield, Middleton & the Dales Way

The path now closely **follows the river** and it is difficult to believe that this rough track was once the only road between Ilkley and Addingham. Having crossed a meadow at Cocken End the path becomes a road (Ilkley Old Road). After about 500m, **turn right** and continue along Old Lane to Smithy Greaves. Note a blue plaque on the first old cottage (See Walk 4 for details).

Beyond the mill cottages, the path narrows but then opens up again to follow Low Mill Lane. The Old Rectory, standing proud on the right, gives an idea of the status of the Rector in years gone by. The current, more modest, Rectory is on the left before the Old Rectory gates.

The path goes **down the steps on the right** and up through a gate into the churchyard. This is the Parish Church of St Peter (see Walk 4 for details). Again, note the blue plaque on the wall outside the main gate.

After reaching the main drive, **bear right over a small bridge** to come out at the North Street and Church Street junction. Continue along Church Street and back to the start point at the **Memorial Hall**.

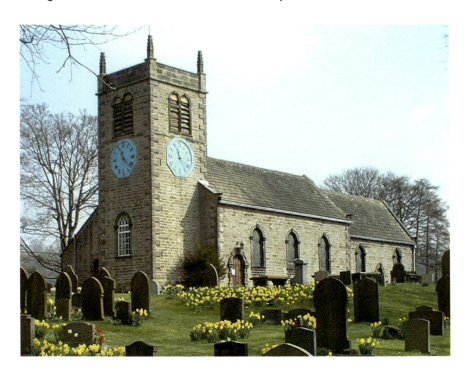

St Peter's Church

Walk 4
The Addingham Blue Plaques Trail
(Note: At the time of going to press plaques 1, 3 and 5 have yet to be positioned. It is hoped that they will all be in place by the end of 2018)

Start & Finish: Addingham Memorial Hall, Main Street, Addingham, LS29 0LZ, SE 079 497
Full walk: 7½ miles (12 km)
Medium walk: 4½ miles (7 km) (excluding Farfield Meeting House)
Short walk: 3¾ miles (6 km) (excluding Farfield and the Band 'Oil)

Summary:

Addingham Civic Society and Parish Council are erecting thirteen blue plaques on buildings around the village to commemorate notable people, buildings or events. These are in addition to two bronze plaques which were erected in the 1990s.

The full walk passes all the plaques, and also passes many other places of interest in the village (see map overleaf). The following pages include more historical information than could be written on the plaques themselves.

The going is easy, mainly along roads but including some footpaths where suitable footwear is needed.

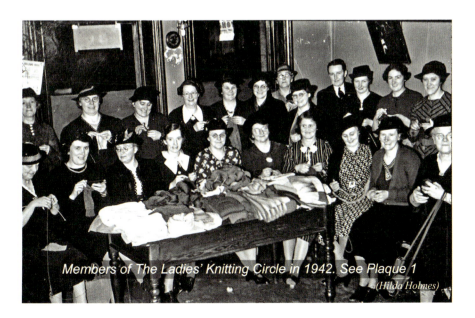
Members of The Ladies' Knitting Circle in 1942. See Plaque 1
(Hilda Holmes)

Walk 4: The Blue Plaques Trail

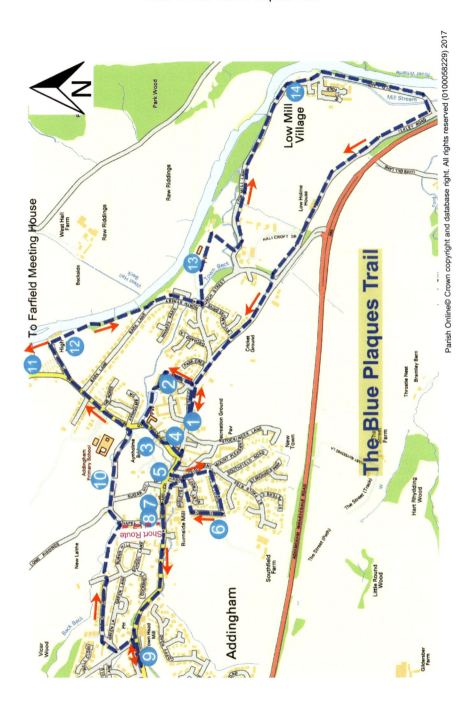

The Trail

Plaque 1: The Women's Knitting Circle & The Memorial Hall

The first plaque on this trail is at the start point, the Memorial Hall. This commemorates the ladies of the Addingham Knitting Circle and their part in the purchase of The Memorial Hall for the village.

During the Second World War, ladies across the country set up knitting circles, with the slogan: **'if you can knit – you can do your bit'**, and they knitted for the Army, Navy, Air Force & ARP (Air Raid Precautions) workers. The Women's Knitting Circle in Addingham (shown on p29 in 1942) was a very committed group and as a result of their efforts over 500 articles were knitted, with every member of His Majesty's forces from Addingham being supplied with a pullover, scarf, balaclava, two or three pairs of socks and gloves/mittens. Even Russians on the Eastern Front benefited from their knitting and, at the same time, they were aiming to raise money for a memorial to the men and women of Addingham who had sacrificed so much for their homes and country. It was decided that the memorial should take the form of a village hall and the Primitive Methodist Chapel, which had closed in about 1955, was available. After much fund-raising, and with the help of generous bequests, the chapel was bought, converted, and has been developed over the years to provide the village with a popular meeting and social place for present and future generations. It is a fine tribute to the young men who gave their lives during the war, being ideally placed next to the War Memorial (the above is from *Addingham in the Second World War*, where there is more about those times).

Leave the Memorial Hall, cross Main Street, **go right**, past the War Memorial and **turn left** down Sawmill Lane beside the Co-op food store. This area used to be called Cross End (hence 'Cross End Fold' on the left)

Plaque 2: William Brear

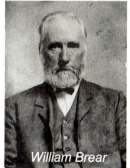
William Brear

At the end of Sawmill Lane, the second Blue Plaque is on Low House (on the corner, left), commemorating William Brear who lived here and started the sawmill business opposite in 1860. His family continued to run it, as William Brear & Sons, until it closed in 2001. The plaque also reminds us that William Brear was a founding member of the Addingham

Parish Council on which he, and other members of his family, notably his son Job Brear, served for a total of 100 years, as well as being active supporters of Mount Hermon Chapel.

The sawmill business occupied a building which was re-built as the apartment block on the right. It was originally built by Anthony Fentiman in about 1796 for his water powered textile mill. This firm closed in the 1850s, following which it was taken by William Brear.

Low House is one of the oldest houses in Addingham with a date stone over the door of 1675 and an internal cartouche dated 1663. Previous to it being bought by the Brears in 1912 it had been occupied by the village doctor and had a special little window through which he handed out the medicines!

Continue through the mill yard and **up the footpath** on the left at the end. This leads past the mill dam (pond) used to supply the original mill waterwheel and fed from under Bolton Road by Town Beck and, originally, Back Beck. **Cross Bolton Road (with great care),** and Town Beck, then **turn left** on the footpath bordering Manor Garth.

Plaque 3: The Rookery

The buildings immediately in front are The Rookery. They were built by John Cockshott in about 1805 as two rows of small, back-to-back, houses with an upper-storey loomshop added across the (right-hand) end, before 1817, for hand-loom weaving. Built in the midst of the textile industry boom, The Rookery saw Adding-

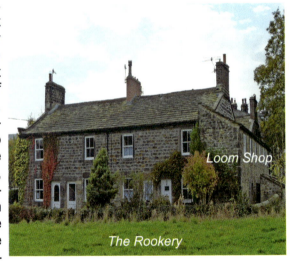

Loom Shop

The Rookery

ham expand greatly from being a small farming community in the mid-18th century to a busy textile manufacturing township 100 years later. The loomshop now only extends across the first row of cottages - the rest having been demolished. Beneath it were the 'tippler' toilets for the cottagers. The name 'The Rookery' has been applied to a number of similar buildings, where people lived (almost) as close together as rooks in a rookery! The back-to-back cottages are now knocked through to make larger homes.

Walk 4: The Blue Plaques Trail

After passing The Rookery, **cross** Bolton Road and continue **down** to Main Street.

Plaque 4: William Kendall Gale - Mount Hermon

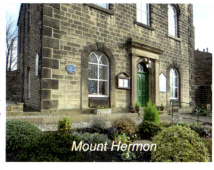
Mount Hermon

On the left corner, facing Main Street, is Mount Hermon Wesleyan Reform Church which has our next blue plaque. This commemorates Pastor William Kendall Gale who, as a student, did good work and greatly helped in raising funds for a planned extensive renovation of the chapel. In 1900 he left to join the Congregational Ministry and in 1908, with his wife the former Edith Gaunt, of Ilkley, went to Madagascar for the London Missionary Society, establishing over 250 churches and many schools in that country. He wrote that '*I regard my pastorate at Mount Hermon as one of the great and happy times of my Ministerial life and am very grateful for the opportunity the church gave me to preach the gospel of Christ and fulfil my call*'.

The chapel was built in 1861 as one of three Methodist chapels in the village - the others being the Primitive Methodist Chapel, which is now the Memorial Hall, and the Wesleyan Methodist Chapel at the top of Chapel Street, which is now housing. The present Methodist Church is in the former school building.

From Mount Hermon, **cross** Bolton Road and **continue up** Main Street, past The Crown, built in 1769, to the lane on the right which leads to Manor Garth.

Plaque 5: The Manor House

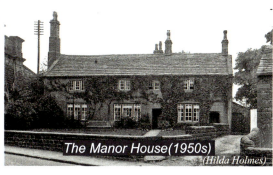
The Manor House(1950s)
(Hilda Holmes)

The house on the left is the Manor House. This has changed greatly over the years, particularly because the front wall was rebuilt in the 19th century, but it has an ancient history. Surveys of the basic structure show that it might date from as early as 1450 but it was most likely built about 1500. Richard and Mary Smith, then Lord and Lady of the Manor, were living in the Manor House in the 1770s and their initials are inscribed on an extension at the back of the house

Walk 4: The Blue Plaques Trail

which was built for them in 1774. The former barns on the other side of the lane are also of a similar age. A striking feature of the Manor House is the chimney at the west (Sugar Hill) end which was extended twice after the railway bridge was built close to the house to improve the draught (*see the 1950s photo p33, showing the railway on the extreme left*).

Richard Smith became Lord of the Manor in 1774 and left an interesting diary of his life. One entry mentions that he walked round his land with a pocket full of acorns (or, as he wrote, 'ackhorns') which he planted in hedges. The oak tree flourishing on Manor Garth near Back Beck Lane is about 200 years old and could well have grown from one of these acorns.

From the Manor House, **cross** Main Street and go **up Old Station Way**. Bear **right** across the grass meadow area and turn **right** along Southfield Lane to the end. **Facing,** at the junction with Southfield Terrace, is Blue Plaque 6 (on the end house).

Plaque 6: Soldiers of WW1

This plaque commemorates all the 414 Addingham men who served in the First World War, 1914-18, of which 83 died. The choice of Southfield Terrace is because, from this row of houses alone, 30 men served and 7 of those never returned. This plaque was unveiled by Robin Ellis, the great-nephew of Charles and William James Ellis, brothers who both lost their lives during the Great War. See *'We Who Served...'* for more details.

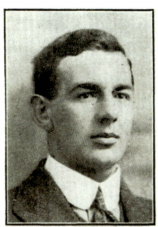
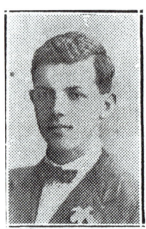

The Ellis Brothers - Charles on the left and William James on the right

Continue down Southfield Terrace, **along** the footpath at the bottom, **down** the steps and then **left, down** to George Street. At the far end of George Street, **re-cross** Main Street to the **Old School**.

Plaque 7: The Old School

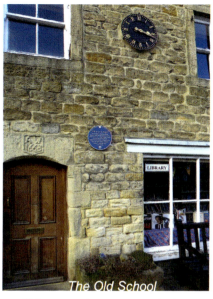
The Old School

This plaque commemorates the building which has been at the heart of the village community for many years. The Old School was built in 1668, as a single-storey cottage, by Anthony Ward (hence the 'AW 1668' datestone). It was later bought by the village as a school and, as the village expanded, was rebuilt with a second storey in 1805. The upper room continued to be used as a school until the Methodist and National (C of E) schools were opened later in the 19th century. The lower rooms were used variously as cottages for the poor, infants' school, village gaol, shops, a barber's and now the village library. When no longer needed as a school, the upper room became, and still is, a function room and Parish Council chamber. **Continue up** Main Street, passing The Swan and the shops to 88 Main Street, on the **right**.

Plaque 8 (bronze): John Cockshott, 88 Main Street

This is one of two *bronze* plaques (the other is on the Old School) which were erected by the Civic Society in the 1990s.

The house was built for John & Martha Cockshott in 1748 and the datestone (right) shows their initials. Like many others of this period in the village, it was built by the local builder and stone mason Joshua Breare. John Cockshott was one of several generations of the family engaged in the textile industry who, between them, built the loomshop in Chapel Street, The Rookery (see Plaque 3) and the impressive 'Piece Hall' opposite.

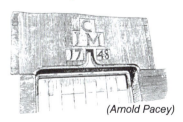
(Arnold Pacey)

This was built by Martin and Samuel Cockshott as a warehouse to which hand-loom weavers would bring their 'pieces' of cloth for sale. In fact, as machine weaving took over, it soon became redundant. It was used as a grocer's shop and then continued as a butcher's until the 1980s. See *'Addingham Houses 1750 - 1850'* for more details.

Walk 4: The Blue Plaques Trail

The next Blue Plaque is on Silsden Road but, if you wish to leave that for later, **take the shorter route by turning right** up Chapel Street to re-join the trail at the top. On the way, you will see Cockshott's Large Loom Shop (built 1806) on the left, the former 'High' School (now the Methodist Church) and the old Methodist Chapel (built 1778) on the right, past the graveyard. **Go to lower down on this page.**

For the full trail, continue up Main Street to the Craven Heifer and **fork left** up Silsden Road. The first building on the left is The Band 'Oil ('Ole or 'Oile, meaning Hole).

Plaque 9: The Band 'Oil

This building was built by the village in about 1686 as a poor house (the original 'Council House'). Originally a two room cottage, the building was later used by the Addingham band, hence the name, but was lived in until the 20th century. It then became ruinous until, in 2007, two villagers, with support from the Parish Council, re-built it for use as a smallholding.

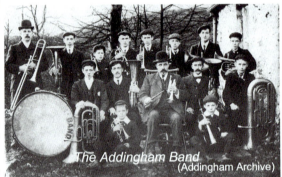
The Addingham Band
(Addingham Archive)

Return down Silsden Road, **cross** Main Street and **go up** Skipton Road to The Green. **Turn right** and then **left** along School Lane, **continuing** well down the lane to a **footpath on the left** where the lane bends right. This path passes chicken-runs beside the beck. At the end **(the short walk re-joins here, on Chapel Street),** continue along Back Beck Lane to the prominent railway bridge.

Plaque 10: Railway Bridge No.55

This is the only railway bridge in the village still looking as it did when the Ilkley to Skipton railway ran through the village. The railway followed the Ilkley Road, crossing it twice, before reaching Addingham station, which was more-or-less on the site of Southfield House on Mount Pleasant (photo p48). The railway crossed Main Street by a bridge at Sugar Hill Green (see photo opposite, top) and then kept close to Bolton Road on its way to Bolton Abbey, crossing Lob Ghyll viaduct (see p15).

The railway must have transformed the lives of people who had only horse-drawn transport up to this time and, even though the early

Walk 4: The Blue Plaques Trail

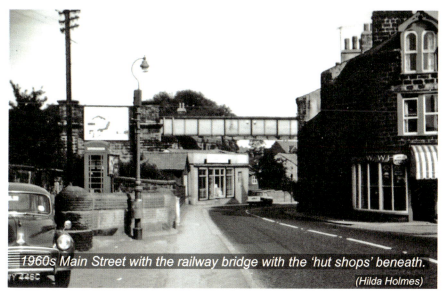

1960s Main Street with the railway bridge with the 'hut shops' beneath.
(Hilda Holmes)

trains travelled a lot slower than now, they then had access to a rapidly expanding network of tracks covering the country.

Continue past the school and turn **left** up Bolton Road, cross Bark Lane and **turn right**, down High Mill Lane to High Mill.

Here there are **two options - for the full walk, turn left** and follow the river bank (The Dales Way footpath) for about 1½ miles (2½ km) until reaching Bolton Road again at Farfield (this is the reverse of the latter part of Walk 1). **Cross** the road **(with care)** and the building beside the road is the Farfield Meeting House.

Plaque 11: The Farfield Meeting House

This is one of the earliest Quaker meeting houses, being dated 1689 which is soon after the Act of Toleration first allowed the Quakers to meet. The land was given to the Society of Friends by Anthony Myers of nearby Farfield Hall as early as 1666. He and other members of the Myers family are buried in the graveyard in stone tombs, which is unusual for the Quakers whose graves are normally unmarked. Another prominent local Quaker was Joshua Dawson (see Plaque 12 below).

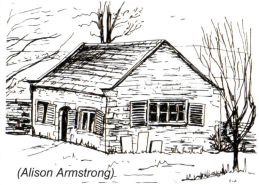

(Alison Armstrong)

37

Walk 4: The Blue Plaques Trail

The Meeting House is now only used a few times a year for Quaker meetings and is owned by the Historic Chapels Trust, cared for by local people. It is open every day and makes an interesting visit.

For the shorter walk, turn right at High Mill, (or after returning along the river from Farfield, keep straight ahead), and go through the car park to the Dawson Crossley field.

Plaque 12: The Dawson Crossley Field

This field and the adjacent river bank, otherwise known as 'The Mill, or Milne, Close', was given by John Crossley and Joshua Dawson to the Overseers of the Poor of Addingham in 1685-6. In the deed for this land, Joshua Dawson decrees ......"that the yearly Rent issue and profits of the said Close let by the said respective Overseers as aforesaid given and distributed according to their discretions to the most indigent and poorest of the poore of the Parish of Addingham...."

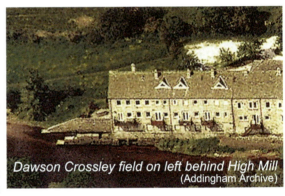
Dawson Crossley field on left behind High Mill
(Addingham Archive)

The field is now the property of the Addingham United Charity but rented by the Parish Council for the free use of all, and it is a pleasant place for a picnic or a bit of fishing.

From the Dawson Crossley plaque, **continue** through the field and **along** the river bank to the steps above the Suspension Bridge. From the top of the steps go **down North Street** and turn **left** just before the junction with Church Street to go into the church field. **Continue** up to the Parish Church gate.

Plaque 13: The Parish Church of St Peter

This plaque commemorates the fact that this has been a place of Christian worship for over a thousand years and was a place of refuge for Archbishop Wulfere of York who fled here in AD 867 from the Viking invasion.

The first Church building was built in the 12th century, possibly on a site of Pagan worship, and was probably of simple wooden construction. In the 15th century this was replaced by a stone building, parts of which, including the north aisle, still survive. The south wall was re-built, and the tower added, in the 18th century to make the building that we see today.

Walk 4: The Blue Plaques Trail

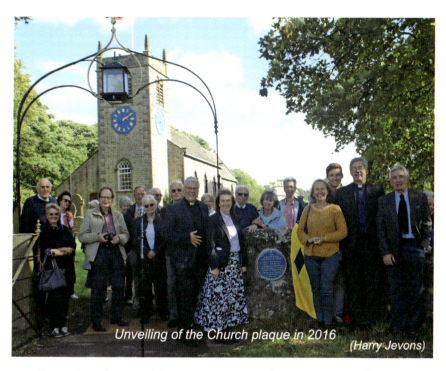
Unveiling of the Church plaque in 2016 (Harry Jevons)

From the plaque at the gateway, **continue** up to the Church and have a look round it (it is usually open) before **continuing** through the churchyard to a **gate on the right**. Go down to the little Moorside Bridge over the beck and **up** the steps to, and **left along**, Low Mill Lane. This was the main access to Low Mill from the village when the mill was working but the last part is now pedestrian only so it is a nice quiet lane beside the river. On reaching the mill cottages **continue**

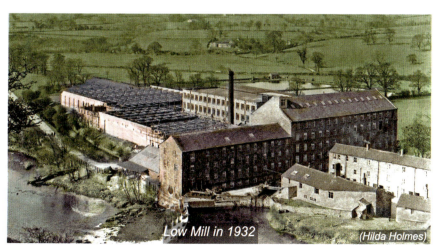
Low Mill in 1932 (Hilda Holmes)

Walk 4: The Blue Plaques Trail

up to the **last cottage** on the right before Holme Ings, where the Penny Hole plaque can be seen on the porch.

Plaque 14: The Low Mill Penny Hole

This **final plaque** on the trail commemorates Low Mill and the fact that this cottage was the mill gatekeeper's home (photo below). He had responsibility for fining millworkers one penny if they were late for work, hence the name.

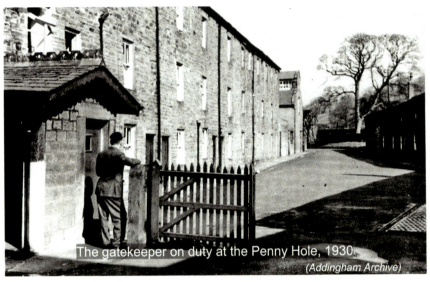
The gatekeeper on duty at the Penny Hole, 1930.
(Addingham Archive)

Low Mill was built in 1787 and became the largest mill in Addingham. In 1826 it was the scene of a riot when 'Luddite' workers from Lancashire, fearing the threat to their jobs posed by the new power driven machinery ordered for the mill, marched to Addingham, led by 'Gurt Bill' from Cowling. They were initially repelled but it required the help of the Yorkshire Hussars, from Leeds, to finally restore order.

The mill was most famously run by members of the Cunliffe-Lister family and was the first successful worsted spinning mill. Various other textile materials were produced here, including silk and velvet, but during the Second World War it was taken over for the production of carburettors for Spitfire and other warplanes.

The workers' cottages were renovated as Low Mill Village in 1985 and the last use of the mill, for wool scouring, ended early this century.

From the Penny Hole, **continue along Old Lane,** pausing to look at the weir on the left, and turn **right** at the T-junction along Ilkley Old Road. At the junction with Church Street, **cross with care** and **continue** along Ilkley Road, and then Main Street, back to the **Memorial Hall.**

Walk 5
Netherwood House, Heber's Ghyll and the Moor Edge

Start & Finish: Memorial Hall, Main Street, Addingham LS29 0LZ, SE 079 497
Full walk: Approx. 6½m (10½ km)
Short walk: 4m (6½ km)
Height gain: 928ft (282m)

Summary:

Starting from Addingham, the walk climbs in a south-easterly direction up the Addingham Moorside meadows to the edge of Ilkley, crosses the bridges up over the tumbling waters of Heber's Ghyll, continues along the breezy edge of the moor for 1½ miles (2½ km), and then back down to the village. A shorter option stays below the edge of the High Moor but still has fine views.

The going is moderate up the Moorside meadows, the climb steeper up Heber's Ghyll, but the uphill section along the moor edge is more gentle. The first part downhill is rocky through the millstone quarry but the following downhill path through meadows is much easier.

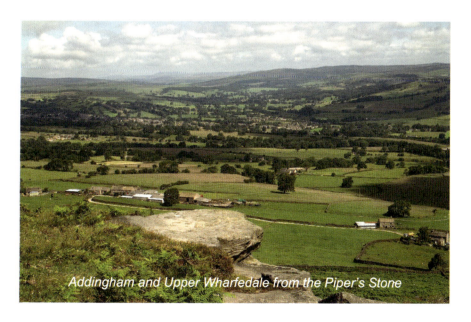
Addingham and Upper Wharfedale from the Piper's Stone

Walk 5: Netherwood, Heber's Ghyll & the Moor Edge

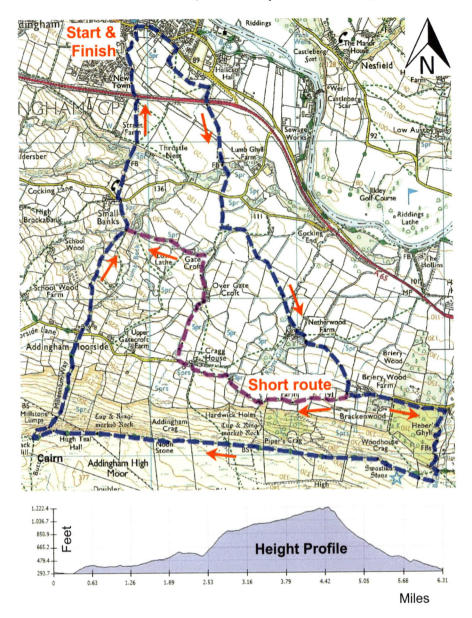

The Walk

From the Memorial Hall, **go right,** down Main Street, to the Cricket Field, turn **right** up the drive to the Pavilion, **left** to the metal gate and continue **straight** along the fence before heading for the gap in the row of trees ahead. Continue **slightly left** to a stile, preceded by a small stream, then **right** up to and across the bypass (A65).

42

Walk 5: Netherwood, Heber's Ghyll & the Moor Edge

From the other side of the road, bear **slightly left** to a white gate and then follow the fence to a stile in the corner. Now head for the **left hand** end of the length of stone wall, **slightly left** to the path down the edge of Lumb Ghyll Wood and left to the bridge across Lumb Beck. This wood is carpeted with bluebells in May. Walk up through the wood (see the Introduction for what to look out for in woods) to the top stile and then **slightly right** to the road (Cocking Lane).

Cross the road and **go up** the drive opposite to the ruins of Plumtree Banks Barn on the left. The area around the barn has been surveyed and found to have evidence of medieval timber buildings and 'ridge and furrow', some of which shows as S-shaped furrows indicating ploughing by oxen.

Just after the ruins **turn left** at the waymarks, on a tree and post, down to, and then **across** Hall Gill beck. Just below here the water in this beck was harnessed, perhaps in the 14th century, to power a furnace and forge for smelting and working iron. Ironstones, mined from nearby shales, were smelted using charcoal fuel produced from the surrounding woodland. Waste slag from these workings can still be found.

After crossing the beck, **follow the fence** round to the **right**, over a wall stile and **diagonally left** across the field, towards the clump of trees, to a metal gate. From the following stile, it's **straight across** the field to find a **low waymark** (right of a large tree) leading to a stone slab bridge across the beck. Go **left** through the field gate and then **bear right** to another gate to enter the grounds of Netherwood House. This was once owned by Mr Greenwood, a prominent Methodist, who gave a croft to the Addingham Wesleyan Methodist Chapel for use as the graveyard, where he lies in a prominent mausoleum. More recently, it was owned by the late Peter Marshall whose philanthropy helped many local organisations. **Turn left** along the road and follow it round to the **right** up to a metal field gate on the **left**, just after the entrance drive. When through the gate, **bear slightly left** across the field, heading for a solitary stone gatepost on the skyline. After the following squeeze-stile, go **straight** across the field towards Briery Hill Farm but, after passing the end of a small beck, **bear right** to a waymark on an electricity pole and up to a small **metal gate** in the wall, followed by a second gate.

This marks the point where the main and short routes diverge - the Main Route continues on the next page.

For the short walk, continue **straight on** from the gate to meet a crossing path and **turn right** along it. **Follow** this path up to the top of the field, and over two wall-stiles. **Follow** the fence, then **wall** (on

Walk 5: Netherwood, Heber's Ghyll & the Moor Edge

the left), to a wall-stile in the corner of the field. Take the **gate on the right** in about 50m which leads past Hardwick House Farm and **continue** along the track, passing Hardwick Cottages, to join the metalled road (Moorside Lane) after the next farm, Cragg House. This farmhouse has a fine ogee doorhead dated 1695 but the frontage was much altered in the 18th century by raising the roof and windows.

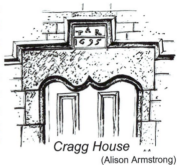

Cragg House
(Alison Armstrong)

About 50m after the farm, turn right at the finger post and **down** the fields, with a hedge and ditch on the left, to a gate in the corner by Over Gatecroft farm (the 'ditch' may actually have been an entrenched packhorse way).

Follow the waymarks left across the drive and then turn **right** down the field, beside the beck, but **bear left** down to the driveway and **turn left** along it, past Gatecroft. After the wall stile, continue along the path across two fields and over Lumb Beck, to go **right** over a small slab bridge. **Here the short route rejoins the full walk (go to p47).**

For the main walk, turn **left** after the second small gate to a wall-stile and across in front of Briery Wood Farm. **Continue** along the drive, and then **keep right** through a gap to follow the footpath behind the roadside wall. After crossing the beck bridge, **turn right** to climb up Heber's Ghyll (photo right). When Ilkley became a popular late Victorian spa resort, many of the place names were tidied up and made more 'romantic'. The spelling 'Ghyll' with its ancient British connotations was substituted for 'Gill'. The stream that ran down from the Moor was renamed Heber's Ghyll, instead of its original (and

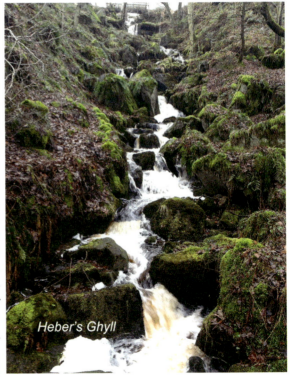

Heber's Ghyll

44

Walk 5: Netherwood, Heber's Ghyll & the Moor Edge

unromantic) Black Beck. Heber's Ghyll was named after Bishop Reginald Heber.

The path and steps up the ghyll are steep but there are frequent benches and the sight of the chaotic, tumbling water (particularly after heavy rain) is spectacular. The path **crosses** the beck, back and forth, over seven wooden bridges and, at the top, turns left to cross the eighth bridge. After this (opposite three benches - another rest?) **turn right up a rocky path** to a crossing, well-surfaced, path. Turn **right** along this, over the beck and through a gate to see the pre-historic Swastika Stone (on the right), a carved stone with a swastika-like design protected by railings. As shown in the photo right, the stone in the foreground is a clearer replica of the actual Swastika stone behind.

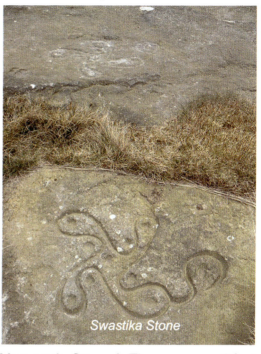
Swastika Stone

This stone is just one of a great abundance of carved stones on the moor; others which are well known include the 'Badger Stone', 'Nebstone' and 'St Margaret's Stones'. These are earthfast boulders, large flat slabs or prominent rocks that have cups, rings and grooves cut into them and are thought to date from either the late Neolithic or the Bronze Age. While some carvings consist of simple cups, others such as the Badger Stone, Hanging Stones and the Panorama Rocks have complex series of patterns (or motifs) combining many different elements. Rombald's Moor has the second highest concentration of ancient carved stones in Europe. There is also a small stone circle known as The Twelve Apostles. Many theories have been put forward as to the significance of these stones, but in reality we have no idea why they were carved. The rock is relatively soft and modern experiments have shown that the carvings can be undertaken quite quickly.

Our route now follows a clearly defined, and much used, path along the edge of Rombald's Moor, of which Ilkley Moor is a part. The moor is said to be named after the local folklore legend of

Walk 5: Netherwood, Heber's Ghyll & the Moor Edge

Rombald the Giant who argued with his wife and threw stones at her across the valley, which still exist as Almscliffe Crag. However, the name is actually likely to be a corruption of Romille, the moors surrounding Skipton having been given to Robert de Romille by William the Conqueror. **The walk continues along** this bracing (if the wind is from the north!) path for about 1½ miles (2½ km), with dramatic views all the way. To the north/north-west is Addingham and, beyond, Wharfedale stretching into the distance; to the east can be seen Ilkley and The Chevin woods above Otley. Piper's Stone, on the right of the path, is a prominent, cup-and-ring marked stone *(see photo on p41)* and, after about a mile, the path passes a large, solitary rock known as the Noon Stone. (This natural stone is mentioned in Paul Bennett's 'Old Stones of Elmet' where it is said that it was 'first described in a boundary perambulation as the 'None' stone in 1579'. It may be representative of sites used for timekeeping

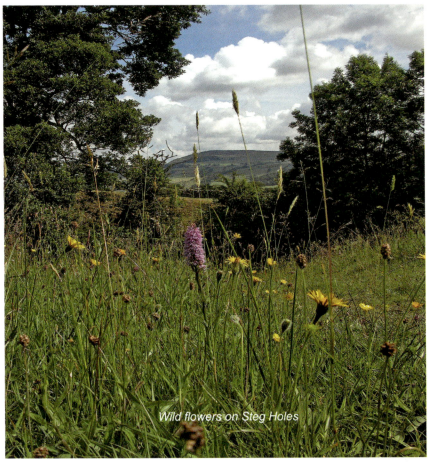
Wild flowers on Steg Holes

Walk 5: Netherwood, Heber's Ghyll & the Moor Edge

or as stones 'over which the noon-day sun appeared'. It marked the boundary between Addingham and Ilkley.)

After about 1½ miles (2½ km) of steady, but moderate, climbing, a well-made cairn marks the top of the route **down** towards Addingham. **Turn right** here and descend the rocky path through the Millstone Lumps quarry where part finished millstones can still be found lower down, though they can be elusive! (See Walk 6.) **After the tall ladder stile** over a 19th century enclosure wall at the edge of the heather covered Addingham High Moor an almost finished millstone can be seen standing in the field on the right (photo, Walk 6). From here, the path is more-or-less **straight down** the hillside to Moorside Lane, near Lumb Beck Farm.

Cross the road and **continue** down the drive beside the farm but **fork left** onto the footpath **before** the sign for Ghyll House Farm. The path goes steeply down the field and up to a gate, **left and right** down to, and over, three wall stiles/gates, passing a caravan park on the left. The last, lumpy, field before a row of trees along Lumb Beck, is a Bradford Wildlife Area known as Steg Holes. This is very colourful with orchids and other wildflowers in the spring and summer (photo opposite). At the bottom of the field, **cross the beck (left)** over a stone slab bridge **(where the shorter walk rejoins)** and continue along the wall and then slightly left across the field to a gate in the wall round the house in the top corner; go round the garden to come out on Cocking Lane which was the main turnpike road between Otley and Colne until 1823. This is the hamlet of Smallbanks, a collection of houses, barns and workshops, mostly dating from the 18th century.

Go a few metres **left** along the road to the footpath **on the right** which goes down to a stile and then **crosses** a small field to a wall-stile and stone steps, known as the Cat Steps, down and then up the sides of a small valley. These old steps would have been used by mill workers walking down to Addingham mills from their farmhouse homes.

From the gate at the top, **continue** slightly left down the field to the gate onto the bypass in the corner of the field. **Cross** the road (more care required) and continue down a green tunnel of holly bushes at the top of Stockinger Lane, over the remains of a railway bridge (Addingham Station used to be on the left here, more or less on the site of Southfield House in Mount Pleasant - photo overleaf) to the football field. Turn right in front of the pavilion and down to the **Memorial Hall** start point.

Walk 5: Netherwood, Heber's Ghyll & the Moor Edge

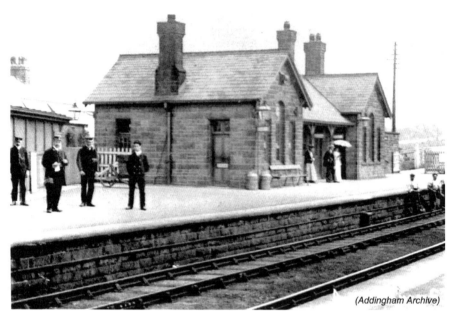

(Addingham Archive)

Addingham Station in about 1930

Walk 6
Moorside and Millstones

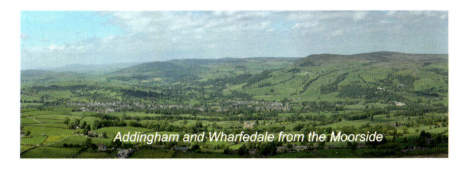
Addingham and Wharfedale from the Moorside

Start & Finish: The Memorial Hall, Main Street, Addingham, LS29 0LZ, SE 079 497.
Full walk: 5 miles (8 km), height gain 830ft (272m).
Shorter walk: 4 miles (6.2 km), height gain 672ft (202m).
Shortest walk: 3 miles (4.8 km), height gain 670ft (202m).

Summary:

The full walk is one of the more energetic in this book but the views over Addingham and up Wharfedale from the edge of the moor, and the sight of the millstone quarry, the Doubler Stones (photo below), and the many traditional farmhouses, make it well worth the effort. The going is fairly gentle uphill across meadows until the Moorside Road is crossed, when it becomes steeper, and can be muddy. The route down is across meadows, steep at first, below Windgate Nick, but then more gentle down to the village. There are two shorter options to give plenty of choice.

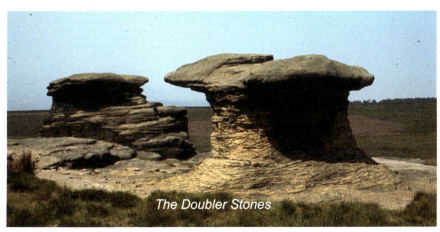
The Doubler Stones

49

Walk 6: Moorside & Millstones

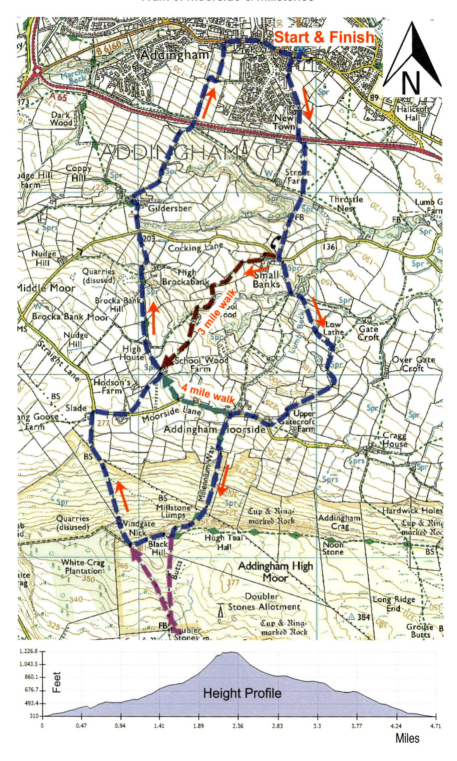

The Walk

From the **Memorial Hall** opposite the Fleece Inn, go **left,** up Main Street and take the **second left** on to Stockinger Lane. The tall houses on the right indicate that they were used by textile workers, with weaving shops above the accommodation. **Continue** up the lane, along a green tunnel of holly bushes to **cross** the Addingham bypass (with care). On the other side, go **very slightly left** across the large Stock Field, where trees indicate the line of former smaller fields. Street Farm, a much altered 18th century farmhouse over to the right, is on the route of the Roman road (see Walk 3).

At the top of the field go through a **wooden gate** and down the Cat Steps into a broad channel cut towards the end of the last ice age (see Introduction, p2).

Throstle Nest, another 18th century farmhouse, can be seen to the left and on the bank opposite the farm, the disturbed ground marks the site of medieval ironstone workings. The path continues **up to** Cocking Lane which is the old turnpike road from Cocken (Cocking) End on Ilkley Road across the open moors to Silsden and on to Colne. Here it passes Smallbanks (photo below), a collection of houses, barns and workshops, also mostly dating from the 18th century.

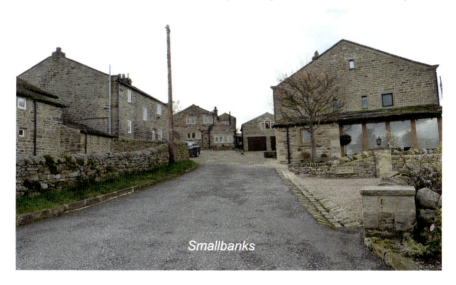
Smallbanks

For the shortest, 3 mile, walk, **turn right** along Cocking Lane and then **bear left** through Smallbanks. After the houses, head **diagonally and gently uphill** across a field to a wall stile. Following the fence line, look for another stile and **turn left** onto a path leading

Walk 6: Moorside & Millstones

into delightful woodland, with a stream, where Cuckoo Nest farmhouse (dated 1758) appears to hide away. Go **over the track** to a small metal gate and continue to head quite **steeply uphill** to the right of Cuckoo Nest and **cross the field** to an obvious wall stile in the far corner. The field beyond leads to **School Wood Farm** where the **longer walks are rejoined**. Turn **right** here for High House **(go to p55)**.

For the longer walks, bear left across Cocking Lane to a small gate in the wall, skirt around a garden to another gate and cross the field to the beck with a stone **slab bridge**. Here turn **left** (east) and cross Lumb Beck and almost immediately, at the end of a short stone wall, **turn right**, bearing steadily and **diagonally** uphill across fields between interesting old stone gateposts.

The barn on the left of the path is Low Laithe, a small field barn which housed 6 cows with hayloft above and a threshing floor. The adjacent fields have been cleared of material from natural landslips that occurred at the end of the ice age. Such landslips, very characteristic of this area, resulted from hillslope collapse during and after the ice melt (see p2). Keep going **steadily uphill** across **several fields**, following waymarks, towards a newly planted copse, including a short, steep section (by which time the copse is on your left), and then **towards** Sunny Bank Farm, on the right, and Moorside Lane.

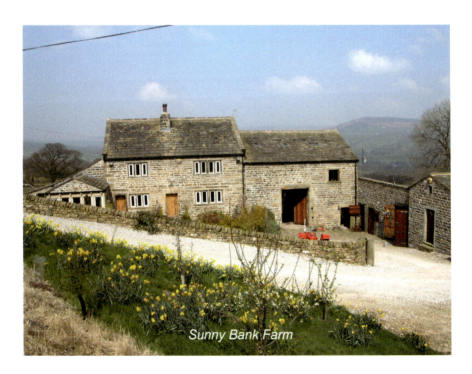
Sunny Bank Farm

Walk 6: Moorside & Millstones

Skirt round to the **left** of Sunny Bank Farm (photo opposite), which dates from about 1740, to Moorside Lane which follows the 800-foot contour and marked the upper limit of crop cultivation in past centuries. The green pastures above the road were once acid moorland but were improved in the 18th century by draining and the application of lime to improve the soil. **Turn right** (west) along the road, passing another 18th century barn. The pecked decoration of the door lintel is seen on many Addingham buildings of about 1790 and may be the work of a local mason called Joshua Breare (see '*Addingham Houses 1750 - 1850*'). **Continue** past Lumb Beck Farm, now entirely rebuilt but incorporating a doorhead dated 1670 and a small window from the original house.

For the shorter 4 mile walk continue along Moorside Lane, **for 500m**, past 18th century houses and Fell Edge Farm (late 18th century) with its unusually large stonework and eaves-level windows. Take the **footpath right**, signed 'Addingham', towards School Wood Farm, where the **full walk** and the **shortest walk are rejoined**, and then High House. **(Go to p55.)**

For the full walk, turn left off Moorside Lane up the **first footpath**, sp 'Millennium Way', which goes **left** over a wall stile and then **straight** up through pasture and moorland to a **high ladder-stile.** An almost finished millstone can be seen in the field to the left (east) just before the ladder stile is reached (photo below). From the 17th century, millstones were manufactured on this hillside, the quarry at the top probably representing the later workings.

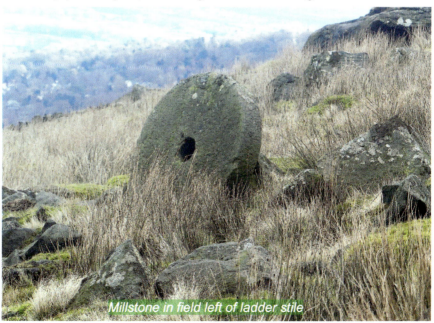
Millstone in field left of ladder stile

Walk 6: Moorside & Millstones

After the stile, bear right and then up through the rocky Millstone Lumps quarry to the cairn at the top of the slope. Fine views can be admired over Addingham to Beamsley Beacon, Simon's Seat, and beyond to Upper Wharfedale, Great Whernside and Buckden Pike to the north-west.

An option now is to take a detour straight across the moor (waymarked 'Silsden Strolls') to see the Doubler Stones (photo on page 49). These spectacular mushroom-shaped stacks of rock are all that is left of the weathered gritstone outcrop. They were formed when the area experienced a cold, tundra-like climate at the end of the ice age.

When returning, fork left soon after the wall (the path is marked by a grassy strip across the heather), heading for a **seat** and small stone pillar on the skyline at Windgate Nick The post (photo right) is a memorial to those killed in a wartime plane crash here (see '*Addingham in World War Two*' for details). **Go to next page.**

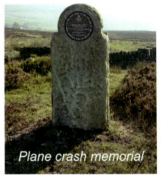
Plane crash memorial

If you are **not going** to the Doubler Stones, **turn right at the cairn and continue** along the moor edge path to the **seat**. In clear weather the distinctive whaleback of Pendle Hill can be seen to the south west. The deep track at Windgate Nick has been created by centuries of use as the route linking Addingham with Silsden and the Aire Valley, passing by the Doubler Stones, Elizabethan coal pits, and 14th century iron working sites in Silsden. 'Johnnie Grey', describing this walk through the Nick from Silsden in 1891, wrote: 'A view of Arcadian loveliness bursts upon the vision, rendered all the more captivating by its complete suddenness. Wharfedale is now revealed in grand array'. This is still very true today and it's well worth sitting on the seat for a while to take it all in. From here it's downhill all the way!

The grassy path **descends** from near the seat (do not take the track) **straight down** to the former farmhouse of Slade, with its fields enclosed within a large circular intake wall. Here **turn right** along Moorside Lane, past Scar Ghyll (18th and 19th century) and take the **footpath, left**, after passing the drive to Hodson's Farm, a laithe-house with attached barn built in the local tradition. **Cross** the field to a gate and continue to School Wood Farm, so named because it was previously owned by Ermysted's School, Skipton. It dates from the early 18th century, but, like many Addingham houses, it was altered later in that century as the farming and textile industry boomed. **Turn left** here over a stile.

The 3 mile and 4 mile walks rejoin the longer one here.

Continue to a wall stile on the left of little High House farm, with its symmetrical frontage and elegant cartouche over the door, which has, for its architectural style, a surprisingly early date of 1697. The back of the house is more traditional in style. **Cross** the small fields ahead, using the wall stiles, with more fine views of Upper Wharfedale, before following the path downhill, **between fences and walls**, with the buildings of High and Low Brocka Bank to the right. Both houses are sheltered by a landslip of sandstone blocks; the lower house is dated 1728. Here the Brocka Bank sandstone has been much quarried, the quarries standing on the open moor until the Enclosure Act of 1873. The fine-grained ganister-like sandstone indicates deposition millions of years ago in a shallow water swamp environment and contrasts with the coarse sandstone of the moors above. Take care on this often muddy, downhill stretch, at the bottom of which **turn left** over the cattle-grid.

Cross Cocking Lane to Gildersber (photo below), an old farmstead first mentioned 800 years ago. The present buildings are

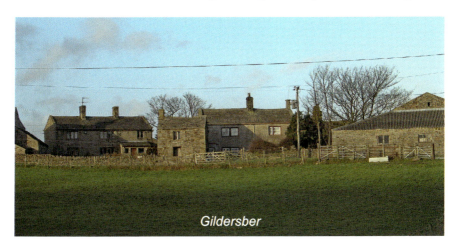
Gildersber

mostly of early 18th century date but the five footpaths which still converge here indicate its former importance. Follow the track to the **left,** then follow the waymarks to turn **immediately right** across a small paddock, **round and through** farm buildings. **Follow the track downhill**, crossing more channels cut by meltwater at the end of the last ice age. Below is the large channel which was crossed previously

Walk 6: Moorside & Millstones

at Cat Steps, followed by the line of the Roman road which is clearly visible here as a raised grassy track with a stone wall on the north side. To the left it is now cut by the Addingham bypass.

Cross over the bypass and **through** a gate into the Southfield, a place name which indicates the site of one of Addingham's large, medieval, open, strip farmed, arable fields. Today the hedgerows of the long thin fields represent former edges of the old ploughed strips. At the bottom of the field **turn right** along a deep hollow lane running west to east, a continuation of Southfield Lane which connects this big open field with the main village.

The route for this walk, however, **goes left** through the gap beside a large oak tree (see p59) and down the field. Dropping down the field, note Burnside Mill (photo below), to the right, then cross the

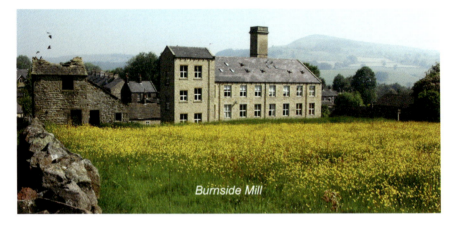

Burnside Mill

Town Beck footbridge and emerge into Main Street. On the left, just after the bridge, note the house with mullioned windows (No.71 Main St), dating from the late 17th century but with an 18th century 'taking-in door' inserted on the first floor so that yarn and cloth could be winched in and out.

Proceeding down Main Street, the legacy of the textile industry and its evolution into the machine age during the Industrial Revolution is evident; take note of Burnside Cottages (1811) across the beck, the mill manager's house (c1800) up to the right of Burnside Mill. Inns such as The Swan (early 19th century) sprang up to cater for travellers to the thriving village and the 1777 Lister's barn (No.99), with its external stone staircase, and adjacent houses, some with datestones, point to these late 18th century boom years. The tall houses on the bend, opposite Sugar Hill, also have taking-in doors.

Continuing down Main Street, the walk finishes back at the **Memorial Hall.**

Walk 7
Southfield, Marchup & High Laithe

Start & Finish: Addingham Main Street car park by Beckside Close, LS29 0PD, SE 075 498,
Main walk: about 2¾ miles (4.4 km),
Height gain 209ft (650m)
Shorter walk: 2 miles (3.2 km)

Summary:

This is a short walk round the top half of the village which includes the ancient Southfield, the village nature reserve at Marchup Ghyll and the 'Museum of Gateposts' at High Laithe. The going is easy, in meadows and on public footpaths, though the section alongside the bypass can be muddy when wet and there is a (shallow) ford, so good footwear is needed.

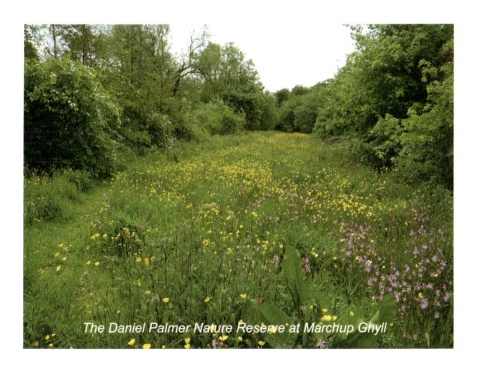

The Daniel Palmer Nature Reserve at Marchup Ghyll

Walk 7: Southfield, Marchup & High Laithe

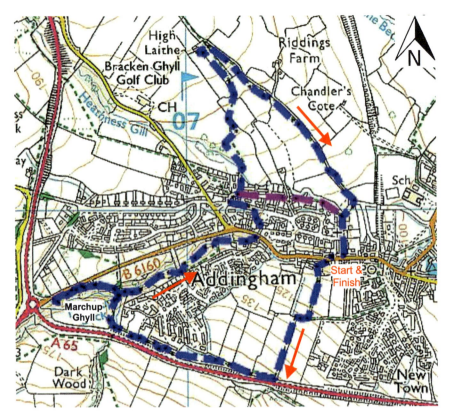

The Walk

Starting from the small car park at Beckside Close on Main Street, cross the **bridge** in the top corner and continue **up the track** to, and through, the little wicket gate which is between two field gates. These gates were once used by the farmers with barns on Main Street to gain access to their fields.

When through the gate, you are in Great Meadow with Newlands Field beyond the wall to your left and Brogden Meadow is the next field to the right. These are known as The Sailor Fields. The small building in Brogden Meadow, partly hidden by a tree, is all that remains of an unsuccessful coal mining operation in the mid-19th century. With increasing mechanisation of industry there was then a growing demand for coal to power steam engines to work the textile mills, and also for domestic use. Here, a group led by Thomas Lister hoped to make their fortune but they found only stone and shale so they were forced 'to give over in consequence of poverty'.

Walk straight up the field beside the wall to the gap beside a large tree. This is now rather narrow and awkward because as the

Walk 7: Southfield, Marchup & High Laithe

200 year old oak has grown it has pushed over the stile and steps in the much older wall (drawing right).

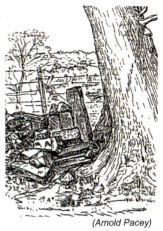
(Arnold Pacey)

Climb over this 'crooked' stile with care and turn right along the hollow lane towards another stile at the end. This lane is hollow because the surface was formed by excavation, with the soil piled into a low bank on one side. This was done in the Middle Ages to make a boundary between 'common' arable land – the village's strip-farmed Southfield to the left – and the privately owned fields to the right between here and Main Street. The lane was used to access these strips and there is still a short length of 18th century cobbled and kerbed path through the end stile. Through the field gate on the left just before this stile can be seen evidence of a strip of the field having been separately enclosed. The left-hand gatepost here is 19th century but the right hand one is of an earlier type.

After the stile, **turn left** up the field, alongside the hedge, and at the top of the field, near the bypass, **turn right** (the 'Dales High Way') along the path parallel with the road, under an overhanging hedge. **Continue** through the field but **bear left** to a gate in the top left-hand corner and along **behind** the housing estate. After a field gate, the path drops down to a beck, which is forded using the stony bed, before turning **right** along the hedge. **Note:** This ford is at the top of a small waterfall and is normally shallow, but may test your footwear! On the right here is Street Farm, named after the Roman Road ('The Street') which passes this point (see Walk 8, p68, for details).

At the bottom of the field **go down** the winding steps and then **left** across Marchup Beck by means of the stepping stones (do **not** cross the wooden bridge yet - that comes later). This shady spot where

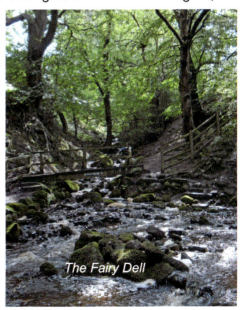
The Fairy Dell

59

Walk 7: Southfield, Marchup & High Laithe

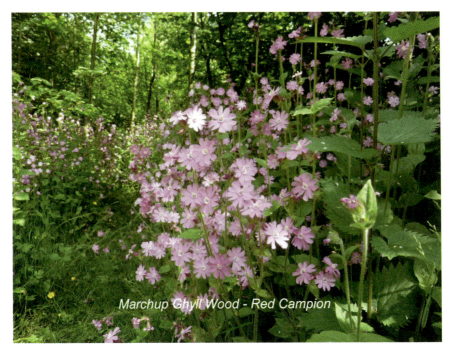
Marchup Ghyll Wood - Red Campion

the two becks meet is known locally as the Fairy Dell (photo p59, look out for the fairies!).

Fork left at the top of the steps to enter the Daniel Palmer Nature Reserve. This area, now known as Marchup Ghyll, was a Victorian landfill site largely composed of ash and glass when the late Cllr Daniel Palmer arranged for it to be covered with soil and planted with trees and wild flowers. That was in 2003 and it is now maturing into a valuable wildlife area, maintained by village volunteers (see photos on p57 & above).

Take the path **up to the woodland** at the top, follow this round the wood and then retrace your steps but go down the little meadow on the **lef**t - this area is ablaze with colourful flowers in season - to the **steps on the right** and back down to the Fairy Dell. Now **cross** the stepping stones and the **wooden bridge** to follow the footpath above the beck to Big Meadow Drive. **Cross** the road and go down to continue following the beck. On the opposite bank, near the bottom of the field, is a building called the 'Band 'Oil' which is marked by a Blue Plaque at the Silsden Road entrance (see Walk 4, p36).

The gate at the bottom leads into the Townhead Trading Estate. This is on the site of Townhead Mill (1966 photo opposite above), one of Addingham's five textile mills, which was built about 1798, originally as a cotton spinning mill but soon converted to producing worsted yarn. The mill burnt down about 1980 and there are now industrial

Walk 7: Southfield, Marchup & High Laithe

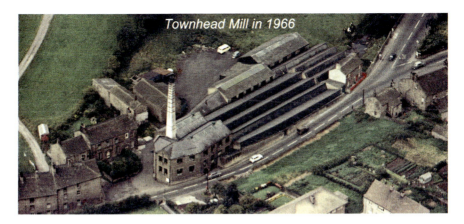
Townhead Mill in 1966

units of various sizes. Situated on the right at the yard entrance, the attractive house, with its classical doorway, was built for the mill manager.

Cross Main Street, **climb** the steps opposite, and **go left** up Green Lane. At The Green, **turn right** along School Lane and **left** along the footpath just after Shearing Path (sp 'Haw Pike'). The Green (originally called 'Robinson's Green') used to be larger but was divided in two when Green Lane was built across it in the 1950s as access to the Council House Estate.

The shorter route continues along School Lane to a footpath on the **left** at the point where the road bends right. This path passes chicken runs beside Back Beck to Chapel Street, where it **rejoins the full walk (go to p62)**.

The full walk now enters the Bracken Hill Golf Course but the hollow area on the left (the 17th green) was Vicar Wood Quarry, earlier known as Spencer's Gill and then as Walker's Gill, one of the many small quarries in the area. Stone from here was used to rebuild the south wall of St Peter's Church and the Church tower in the 18th century, as well as local houses, but was last used for the War memorial, built in 1920. The public footpath **bears right,** crosses a stream and **turns left** to follow the coloured posts up the left-hand hedge, past a large tree, then **across** the fairway (watch out for golf balls!) to a coloured post and gate opposite. **Follow** the path up to a small gate and **continue** up two meadows to a ruined barn at the top, in the field on the left.

This is High Laithe, an 18th century field barn which, like many in Addingham, was enlarged to provide extra accommodation for cattle and hay. Originally, cattle were overwintered in the two byres, or mistals; one is inside the barn and the other under the extended sweep of the roof, and hay was stored above so that it could be fed

Walk 7: Southfield, Marchup & High Laithe

to the cattle from the centre of the barn. Opposite the wide cart entrance is a small 'winnowing door' in the back wall. As crops such as barley and oats were threshed on the stone floor the draught from

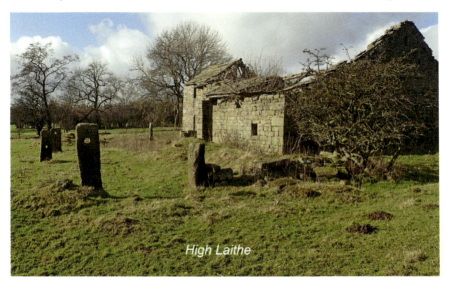
High Laithe

the opened doors separated the grain from the chaff (photo above). Near the barn is a remarkable collection of gateposts (once referred to as a 'Museum of Gateposts') which may be older than the barn as the square holes in them were made to hold crooks of timber which hinged the gate. This method was used when iron was in short supply.

This point marks a **turning point** - from the barn, **cross** to the high hedge and keep this on the **left,** going down the meadows to a gate at the far, bottom left, corner of the **third field**. The path here joins Long Riddings Lane (behind the hedge) which was probably the medieval road to the village's High Field. Continue down the lane and turn right into Chapel Street. Where this road, shortly, bends left **(the Shorter Route rejoins here)** is the original Wesleyan Methodist Chapel, built in 1778 (now housing) - the present Methodist Church on the right was a school.

Follow Chapel Street down to Main Street and, right, to the **start point.**

Walk 8

Pre-Historic Addingham: Counter Hill and Round Dykes

Start & Finish: Townhead Trading Estate, Main Street, Addingham LS29 0PD, SE 072499
Full walk: 5 miles (8km)
Shorter walk: 3 miles (4¾ km)
Height gain (full walk): 575ft (1750m)

Summary:

There was a lot of pre-historic activity around Addingham - witness all the enigmatic 'cup & ring' stones, and other remains, on Rombald's Moor - and this walk goes through another 'hot spot' on Addingham Low Moor with tumuli, enclosures and the striking Round Dykes earthworks. The walk starts at Townhead Mill trading estate at the top of Main Street, follows Marchup Beck to the Daniel Palmer Nature Reserve at Marchup Ghyll, continuing along Parson's Lane up to Addingham Low Moor, looping back to view Round Dykes and finishing close to Heathness Gill, then back to the village. There is a shorter variation for those with less time or energy. The going is gently uphill to begin with and along tracks, footpaths or across grassy meadows but parts of this walk can get very muddy and it is not recommended in wet weather without suitable footwear.

The Walk

The walk starts from the former Townhead Mill at the top of Main Street which was built about 1798, originally as a cotton spinning mill but soon converted to producing worsted yarn. The mill burnt down about 1980 and is now industrial units. The attractive house, with its classical doorway, situated at the yard entrance, was built for the mill manager and the tall row of three-storey houses below the mill entrance, facing Main Street, illustrates another aspect of

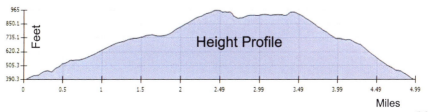

Walk 8: Counter Hill & Round Dykes

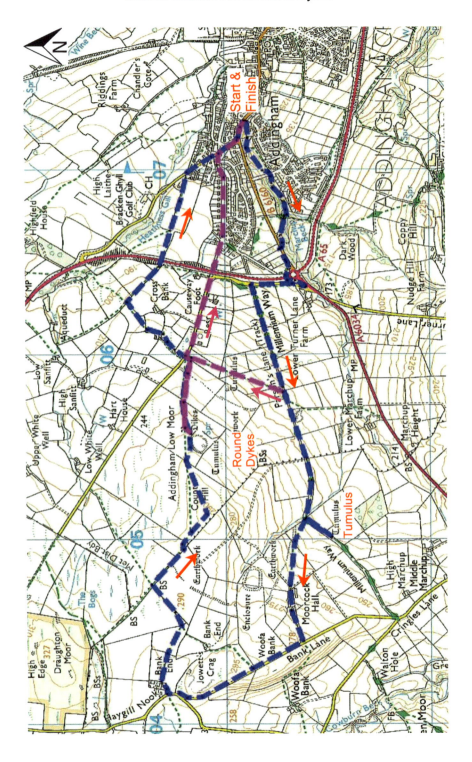

Walk 8: Counter Hill & Round Dykes

Addingham's textile industry in that the top floors housed hand-weaving looms, with housing below. It is known as Independence Row because Baptists worshipped in the end house in the early 19th century.

From the top of the mill yard, **the route follows Marchup Beck**, passing, on the opposite bank, a building now used as a smallholding known as 'The Band 'Oil' (see Walk 4, p36, for details). At the end of the field, **bear left** up to the wall stile and **cross** Big Meadow Drive. This road is built on a dam constructed to prevent storm water in the beck flooding the village – the sluice building can be seen just up-stream.

Continue parallel to the beck and, immediately after the wooden bridge, **turn right** to **cross** Marchup Beck by stepping stones. Fork **left** at the top of the steps into the Daniel Palmer Nature Reserve (see Walk 7 for details). From the top gate, **cross Silsden Road**, up to the roundabout, **cross the bypass** and go **left** and then **right** into Crossbank Road. This road was built when the bypass was constructed (it opened in 1991) to give access to upper Parsons Lane and Moor Lane.

Turn left into Parsons Lane (sp 'Oaktree Farm') which was a track across open heather moor until 1873 when Addingham Low Moor was enclosed with stone field walls and cultivated. Looking back, there is a fine view down the valley to Ilkley and beyond but there will be even better views later in the walk.

For the shorter walk:

Take the footpath right (sp 'Moor Lane 0.5 miles') soon after the farm, and go over the wall stile on the **right** after about 25m. Go **diagonally** across the field to a stile in the right hand top corner of the field, **across** the next, small, field and along the third field to go **left** over the **wall stile** about 20m from the far gate. There are a number of markers inscribed "BCWW" (Bradford Corporation Water Works) which relate to water supply aqueducts built in the last century to convey water from large reservoirs, such as on Barden Moor, to the thirsty industrial town of Bradford.

Climb gently up the field and over another stile into the next field, going **left** at a solitary marker post towards the wire fence to view Round Dykes (description on next page). Return the same way but **turn left** after the second stile and **right down Crossbank Road** to the bypass. **Cross with care**, continue down Moor Lane and right down Skipton Road back to the start point.

For the main walk:
Continue straight up Parsons Lane, through a gate (sp 'Public Bridleway'), where it becomes a green way. Note the old, worn, paving

65

Walk 8: Counter Hill & Round Dykes

stones ('trods') dating from when this was a much-used route into Addingham before Silsden Road was built in the 19th century. After the second gate the route goes over a **wall stile on the right** just after the bend in the track. However, a **small deviation** is suggested to view the pre-historic round tumulus shown below. **For this, continue** on the lane round to the left for about 100m to the tumulus (on the left side of the track) and **return up** the lane and over the wall stile, **now on the left**.

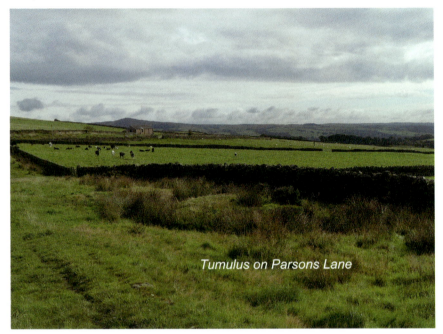
Tumulus on Parsons Lane

From this stile, **go straight across** to another **(rather high!)** wall stile and then slightly left to the gate at the corner of the field, near the farm buildings.
Walk through the farmyard, past the front of Moorcock Hall and up the drive to Bank Lane. **Turn right** up the road, keep right and take the **second footpath (right)** after about ½ mile (Bank End Farm). Walk round in front of the farm, **through** the farm gate and keep close to the wall on the right to another gate. **Continue** parallel to the wall to a wall stile (or use the gate). **Keep straight**, with the wall still on the right, to a ladder stile in the far corner. **Turn right** here, along the wall, which marks the boundary between Addingham and Silsden, to a distant, facing wall stile, about 25m from the corner of the field.

The route now enters a large field enclosing the gentle summit of Counter Hill, ahead, the high point of the area at 885ft (290m). From here the magnificent views in every direction include Embsay Moor

Walk 8: Counter Hill & Round Dykes

(NW); Upper Wharfedale (N) with Simon's Seat and Great Whernside; the Bolton Abbey Estate (NE, beyond Chelker Res.) with the Vale of York and North York Moors in the distance; Beamsley Beacon (E); Rombald's Moor, Ilkley and Otley Chevin (S - SE) and Pendle Hill (SW) all visible on a clear day. Purple heather colours many of these hills in late summer.

From the summit, **walk down** the field in the direction of Beamsley Beacon across the valley, to a fence stile. Follow the wire fence to view **Round Dykes** (photo below) on the right behind the fence. This is a circular earthwork which enclosed a farming settlement, with huts inside the banks and ditches. It dates to the Iron Age, more than 2,000 years ago, when the climate was warmer and drier than today's. Domestic animals kept up here were safe from predators, such as wolves, which inhabited the forest of Wharfedale in the valley below. The site is protected by the Department of the

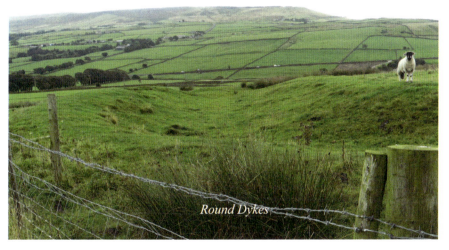
Round Dykes

Environment as a scheduled monument.

Turn left, away from the earthworks, to a solitary wooden signpost in the middle of the field and follow the waymark (right) to a stile. Go down the next field to the electricity pole opposite and over a wall stile at the bottom of a small quarry. Here **turn left** to come out on Crossbank Road, formerly Moor Lane. This runs straight down to Addingham, **as used by the short route if you prefer a more direct route home.**

Crossbank Road follows the course of the Roman road ('The Street') built nearly 2,000 years ago to connect Tadcaster to Ribchester via the forts at Ilkley and Elslack. Part of the original

Walk 8: Counter Hill & Round Dykes

the road if you have time to take another detour. This was the main road to Skipton until about 1803 but its steep inclines were notorious to travellers. According to Harry Speight, writing about 1900, the poet Thomas Grey travelled this road in 1769 and he declared Short Bank (near Skipton) to be the steepest hill he ever saw a road carried over in England. On descending into Addingham, note the number of interesting gateposts cut with a square hole in them. These have been re-used, but probably date from the field enclosures of the 16th or 17th century. The square hole held a wooden crook which hooked around the upright timber of the gate and so hinged it (see sketch right).

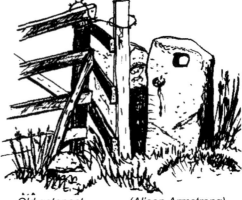

Old gatepost   *(Alison Armstrong)*

To continue on the main route take the footpath across the road, right of the drive to Low Cross Bank Farm which dates from the late 17th century and was the home of some of Addingham's stone masons (there were small quarries nearby). It has typical small windows, and a circular stair turret at the rear.

The path goes round the farm and then **right**, following the wall on the right to a stile in the corner of the field. Here, **turn right** on a crossing footpath and follow the wall on the **right**, through two wall stiles, down to the bypass (Wharfedale Road).

Cross the bypass (with care) and follow the footpath down two fields to Skipton Road. This was built in about 1803 to replace the old, higher, road which is now Crossbank Road (see above). Turn right down the road and round to the left by the Craven Heifer, back to the **start point at Townhead.**

Other books from Addingham Civic Society:

***Addingham – From Brigantes to Bypass* by Kate Mason (1996)**
A definitive history of the village, by local historian, the late Kate Mason

***Addingham Houses 1750 – 1850* by Arnold Pacey (2014)**
Before 1750 Addingham was a small farming community, but during the next 100 years the village was transformed by the coming of the textile industry and the construction of substantial mills and related enterprises. This book describes the houses built, and who built them, during this period.

***We Who Served…, Stories of Addingham and The Great War, 1914-1918* by Catherine Snape (2015)**
From Addingham, a close-knit village of millworkers and farmers, with a population of less than 2,000, over 400 men marched off to fight in the 1914-1918 war. This book describes the experiences of those men and the families they left behind.

***William 'Bill' Bradley, Addingham's Most Inventive Engineer* by Don Barrett & Ian Crawshaw (2016)**
This book describes the life of William Bradley from his birth in 1885 to his death at the great age of 98. Starting as a vehicle repair and servicing mechanic he was also a motorcycle trials rider who designed and built remarkable bikes and he later became a manufacturer of innovative textile industry equipment.

***Main Street Memories; Living and Shopping in 1940s Addingham* by Don Barrett, Beryl Falkingham & Gloria Stitt (2015)**
Present day Addingham is very different to what it was during the Second World War and the 1950s. This book describes the everyday life of two young girls growing up on Main Street during the war and an imaginary shopping trip along Main Street.

***Addingham in World War Two* by Richard Thackrah & Beryl Falkingham (2017)**
This book describes the ways villagers worked for the war effort, has a diary of wartime newspaper reports and details of those who lost their lives in the 1939-45 conflict.

These books are available from Amazon or from the society:
email: *info@addinghamcivicsociety.co.uk*

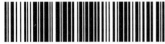

Printed in Great Britain
by Amazon